Patanjali, the patron saint of Yoga, said that mastery combines a balance of science and art. Knowledge of science is like the colors on an artist's palette – the greater the knowledge, the more colors available. The body is the canvas and the Asanas are the art we create.

Scientific Keys | Volume I

Attention: Dislclaimer

Design: Ingrid Patricia Sanchez

Proofreader: Eryn Kirkwood, MA

www.BandhaYoga.com

Printed in China
11 12 13 14 15   10 9 8 7 6 5 4

About the Author

Ray Long

Ray Long MD, FRCSC, is a board certified orthopedic surgeon and the founder of Bandha Yoga. Ray graduated from The University of Michigan Medical School with post-graduate training at Cornell University, McGill University, The University of Montreal, and Florida Orthopedic Institute. He has studied Hatha Yoga for over 20 years, training extensively with B.K.S. Iyengar and other of the world's leading Yoga masters.

Chris Macivor

Chris Macivor is a digital illustrator and the visual director of Bandha Yoga. Chris is a graduate of Etobicoke School of The Arts, Sheridan College, and Seneca College. His work has spanned many genres, from TV and film to videogames and underwater videography.

Contents

Scientific Keys

How To Use This Book

The images in this book are the keys. We present each muscle in the context of its function as an agonist, antagonist, or synergist. Note the interrelated views of the muscle in each of its various representations.

Relax and study one muscle at a time. Actively apply what you have learned by visualizing the muscles as you perform the Asanas. Consciously contract and relax the muscles, as detailed in the images. This will consolidate your knowledge. Review each studied muscle, first at 24 hours and then again at 1 week. In this way, you will master the muscles and integrate them into your Yoga practice.

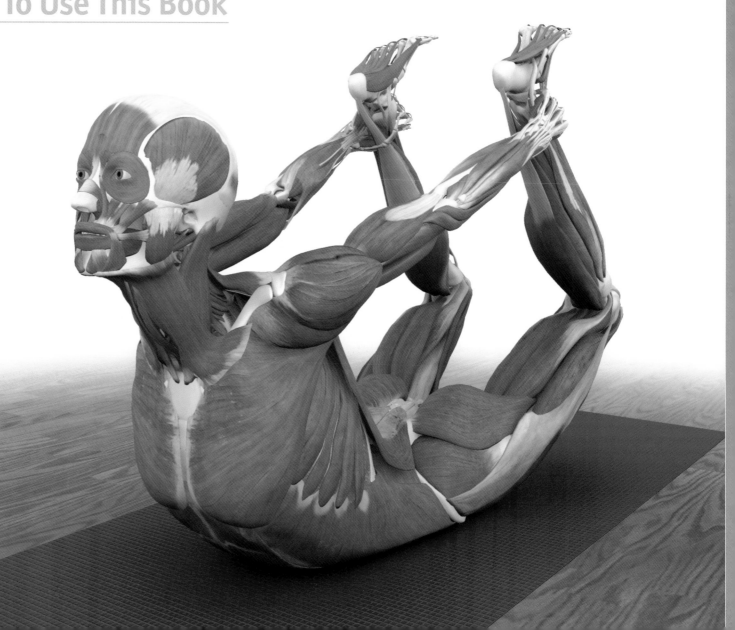

Introduction

Human anatomy and physiology is a vast subject, as is the art of Hatha Yoga. Nevertheless, combining knowledge from both fields is extremely beneficial to the Yoga practitioner. Athletes can improve their performance and experience fewer injuries through a basic understanding of their musculoskeletal system. Similarly, Yoga practitioners can benefit from the application of Western science to their practice development.

It is not necessary to memorize hundreds of muscles and bones to experience the benefits of applying science to Yoga. What is necessary is the functional understanding of a manageable number of key anatomic structures, in their settings, as they relate to Hatha Yoga. Knowledge of these structures can be applied immediately to optimize your practice, break through blockages, and avoid injuries.

This first volume presents key muscles in the context of Hatha Yoga. For practitioners unfamiliar with the Western scientific terminology of the body, the following section, "Fundamentals," is recommended.

Fundamentals

Locations of Structures on the Body

The following terms are used to describe where structures lie in relation to certain landmarks on the body.

Medial:
Closer to the midline of the body

Lateral:
Away from the midline

Proximal:
Closer to the trunk or midline

Distal:
Away from the trunk or midline

Superior:
Above or toward the head

Inferior:
Below or away from the head

Anterior:
Toward the front of the body

Posterior:
Toward the back of the body

Ventral:
On the front of the body

Dorsal:
On the back of the body

Superficial:
Toward the skin

Deep:
Inside the body

Locations on the Body

These images demonstrate the terminology for identifying body locations in Yoga postures. Note that some of the terms are interchangeable. For example, an anterior structure (such as the chest) in Utkatasana is also ventral.

1) **The sternum is medial to the shoulder.**

2) **The shoulder is lateral to the sternum.**

3) **The shoulder is proximal.**

4) **The hand is distal.**

5) **The head is superior to the feet.**

6) **The feet are inferior to the head.**

7) **The chest is anterior to the back.**

8) **The back is posterior to the chest.**

9) **The abdomen is ventral.**

10) **The lumbar region is dorsal.**

11) **The abdominal muscles are superficial.**

12) **The abdominal organs are deep.**

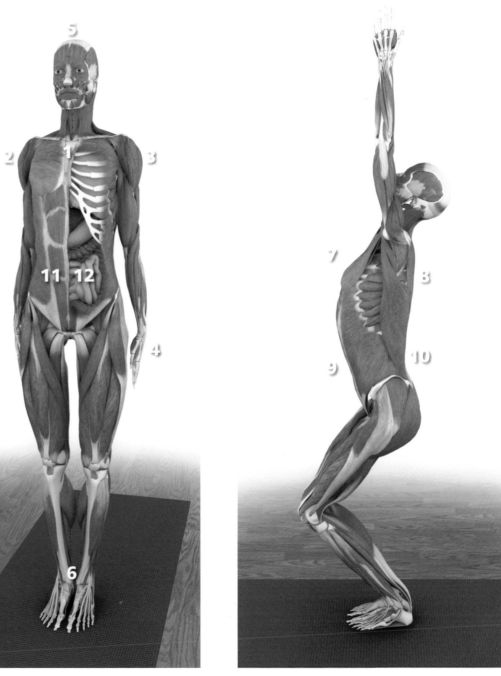

Tadasana

Utkatasana

Skeleton

Bone is the dynamic living tissue that forms the body's structural framework. Bone mass is composed of organic and inorganic materials, including calcium salts and connective tissue, as well as cells and blood vessels within a calcium matrix. This combination gives bone a tensile strength near that of steel, yet it maintains a modicum of elasticity. By aligning the direction of the force of gravity along the major axis of the bones, we can access this strength in Yoga postures.

Regular practice of Yoga is beneficial for your bones because healthy stresses are applied in a variety of unusual directions. This strengthens bones, which remodel in response to stress by depositing layers of calcium into the bone matrix. Like a physiological yin/yang, lack of healthy stress on bones weakens them.

Bones are also the body's reservoir for calcium, critical in a variety of physiological functions, including muscle contraction. The concentration of calcium in the body is tightly regulated through a complex interplay between the skeletal, endocrine, and excretory systems. This involves feedback loops between the parathyroid gland, the kidneys, the intestines, the skin, the liver, and the bones.

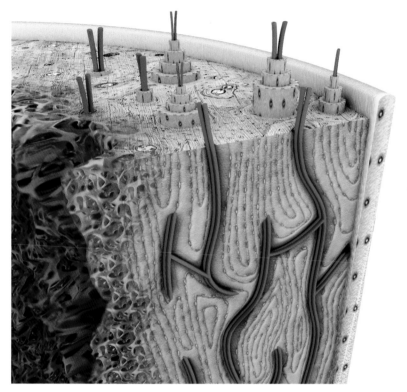

living bone

Bone mass decreases in osteoporosis. This age-related decrease is associated with the loss of estrogen in post-menopausal women. Studies have demonstrated that resistance exercise maintains bone mass. Accordingly, it is reasonable to conclude that the various healthy stresses that Yoga practice applies across the bones may aid in preventing osteoporosis.

The bones of the skeleton link together at the joints and act as levers for the muscles that cross the joints. Consciously contracting and relaxing these skeletal muscles moves the body into the various Yoga postures.

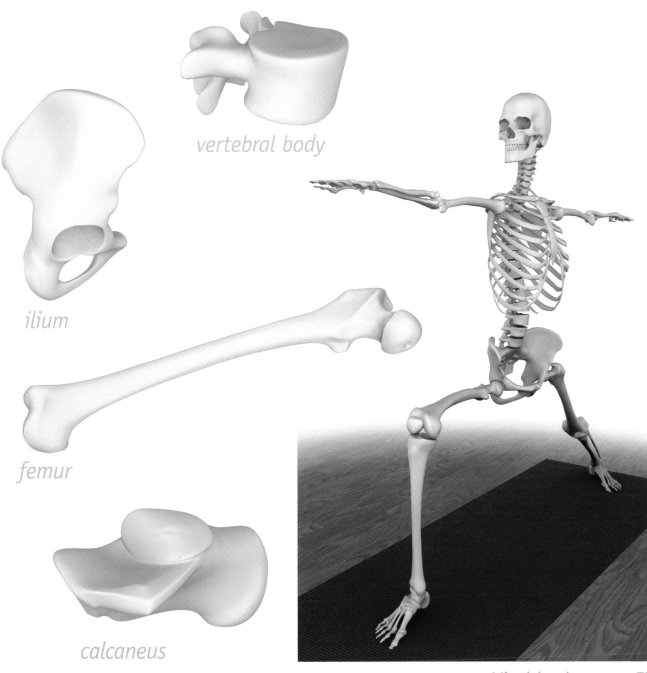

vertebral body

ilium

femur

calcaneus

Virabhadrasana II

Shapes of Bones

The form or shape of a bone reflects its function. Long bones provide leverage, flat bones provide protection and a place for broad muscles to attach, and short bones provide for weight bearing functions.

Yoga accesses each bone's particular potential, using the long bones to leverage the body deeper into postures, the flat bones (and their accompanying core muscles) for stability, and the short vertebral bodies to bear weight. Examples of these bones are illustrated here.

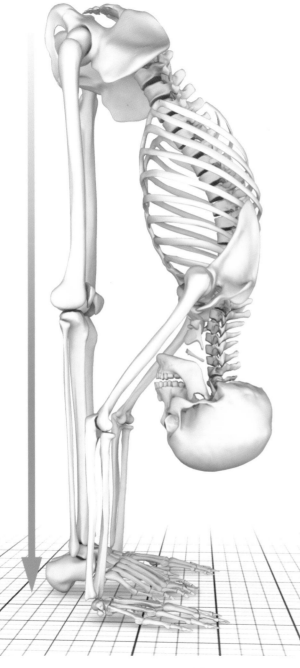

Gravity and the Skeleton

The Sanskrit word for a Yoga pose is Asana. Sanskrit scholars variously translate this word to mean "a comfortable or effortless position." Yoga postures approach effortlessness when we align the long axis of the bones with the direction of gravity. This decreases the muscular force needed to maintain our postures.

For example, in Uttanasana, the force of gravity aligns with the long axis of the femur and tibia bones. Similarly, in Siddhasana the force of gravity aligns with the long axis of the spine.

Use muscular force to bring the bones into a position where they carry the load. Once these positions are attained, muscular force is no longer necessary (or is greatly decreased).

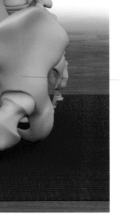

Uttanasana

Siddhasana

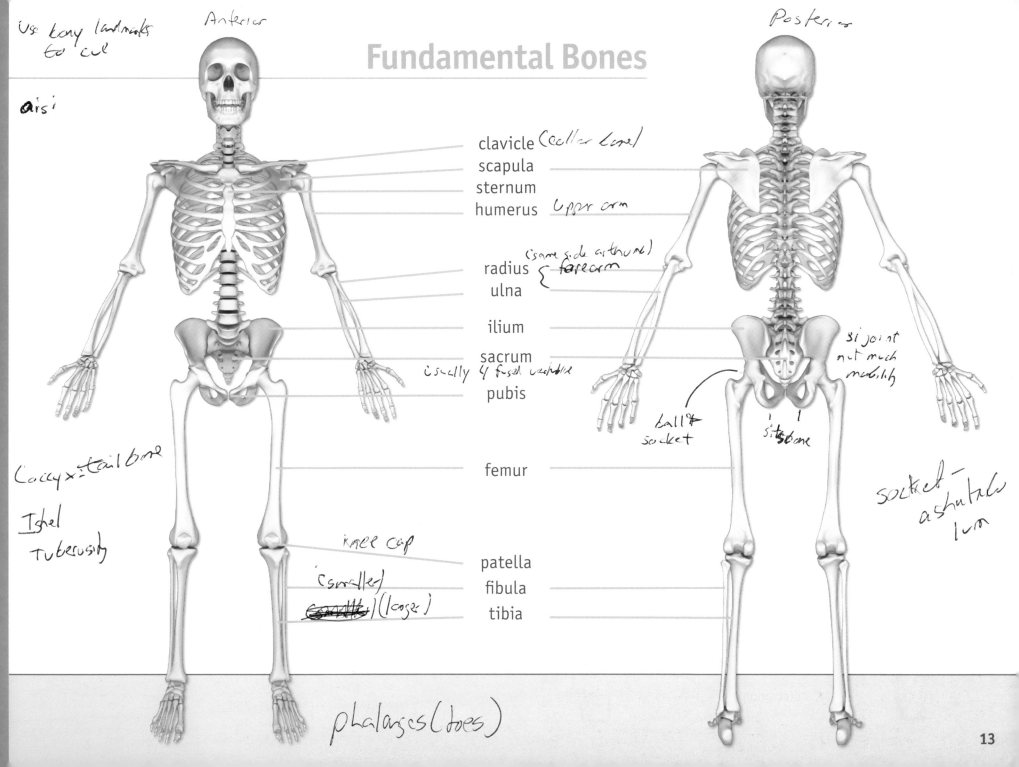

Fundamental Bones

Use bony landmarks to cut

asis

Anterior

Posterior

clavicle (collar bone)
scapula
sternum
humerus — Upper arm

radius {(same side as thumb) forearm
ulna

ilium

sacrum — usually 4 fused vertebra
pubis

si joint not much mobility

ball & socket

sits bone

Coccyx = tail bone
Ishel
Tuberosity

femur

socket — astutule lum

knee cap
patella
(smaller)
fibula
(larger)
tibia

phalanges (toes)

Fundamental Bones

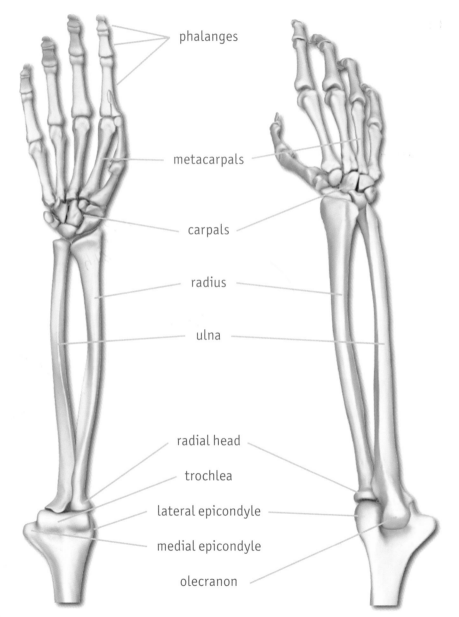

phalanges

metacarpals

carpals

radius

ulna

radial head

trochlea

lateral epicondyle

medial epicondyle

olecranon

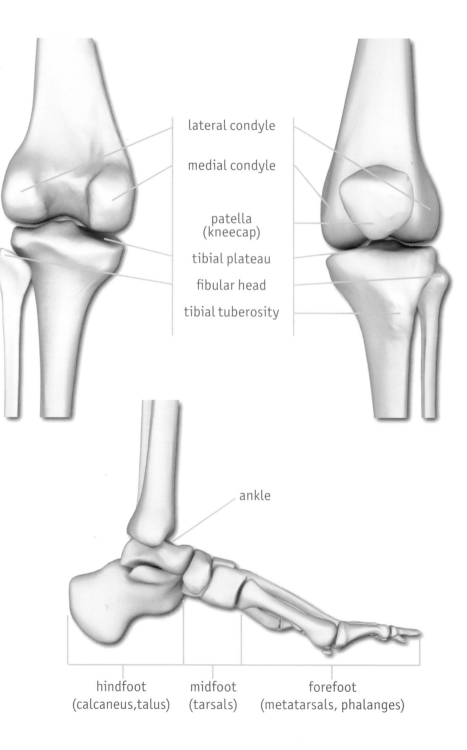

lateral condyle

medial condyle

patella
(kneecap)

tibial plateau

fibular head

tibial tuberosity

ankle

hindfoot
(calcaneus, talus)

midfoot
(tarsals)

forefoot
(metatarsals, phalanges)

Shoulder and Hip

The hips and shoulders are ball and socket joints. Their form reflects their function, in that the deep socket (acetabulum) of the hip is designed to support weight, while the shallow socket (glenoid) of the shoulder is designed to provide maximum range of motion for the arms. Yoga postures balance mobility and stability by increasing the range of motion of the hips and stabilizing the shoulder.

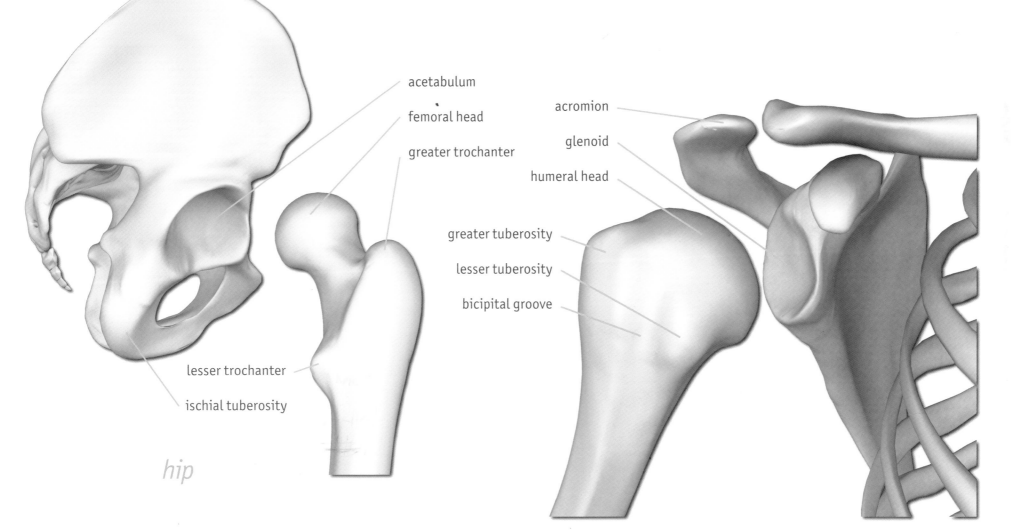

acetabulum

femoral head

greater trochanter

lesser trochanter

ischial tuberosity

hip

acromion

glenoid

humeral head

greater tuberosity

lesser tuberosity

bicipital groove

shoulder

The Axial and Appendicular Skeletons

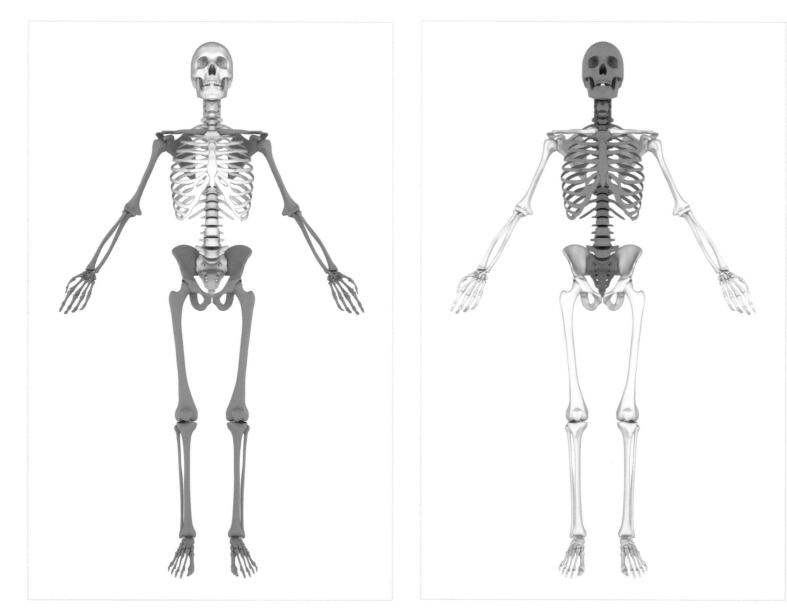

The axial skeleton consists of the spinal column, cranium (skull), and rib cage. The spinal column surrounds and protects the spinal cord, which is the central energy channel, or Sushumna Nadi. It is the axis around which the poses of Yoga revolve. The appendicular skeleton connects us with the world: the lower extremities form our connection to the earth, and the upper extremities, in association with our senses, connect us with each other.

axial skeleton

appendicular skeleton

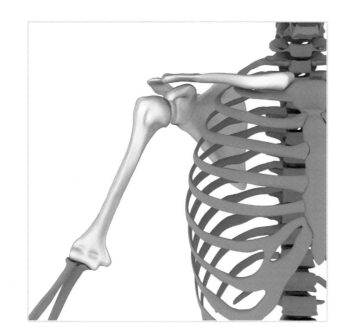

The Shoulder Girdle

The shoulder girdle is the yoke that connects the upper extremities to the axial skeleton. It is the seat of the brachial plexus, a collection of nerves that, in association with the heart, forms the basis for the fourth and fifth Chakras. The shoulder girdle is comprised of the following structures:

· Scapula (shoulder blade)
· Scapulothoracic joint
· Clavicle
· Sternoclavicular and Acromioclavicular joints
· Humerus (upper-arm bone)
· Glenohumeral joint

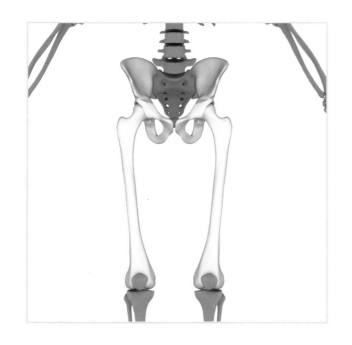

The Pelvic Girdle

The pelvic girdle is the yoke that connects the lower extremities to the axial skeleton. It is the seat of the sacral plexus, a collection of nerves that forms the basis for the first and second Chakras. The pelvic girdle is comprised of the following structures:

· Iliac bones
· Sacroiliac joint
· Femur (thigh bone)
· Hip joint

Connecting the Appendicular and Axial Skeletons

Eka Pada Viparita Dandasana demonstrates connecting the upper and lower appendicular skeletons to create movement in the axial skeleton. Note the inset image demonstrating the stimulation of spinal nerves in this back bend.

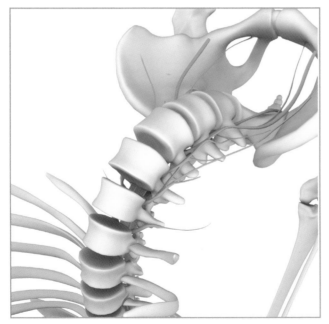

nerve roots in a back bend

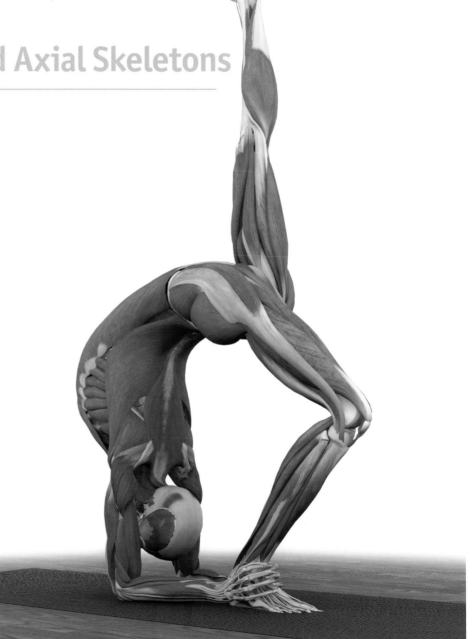

Eka Pada Viparita Dandasana

The Vertebral Column

Between each vertebrae is a squishy disc

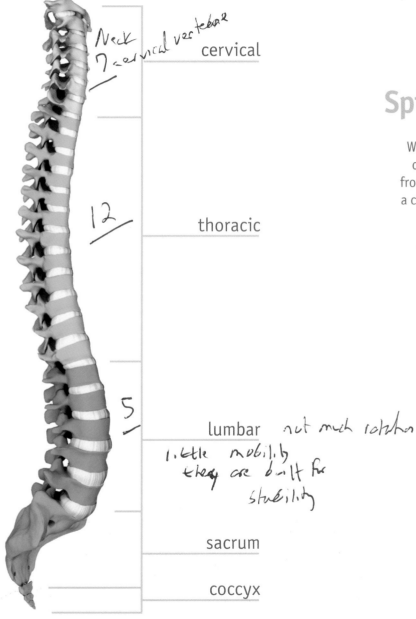

Neck
7 cervical vertebrae

cervical

12

thoracic

5

lumbar *not much rotation*

little mobility they are built for stability

sacrum

coccyx

Spinal Curves

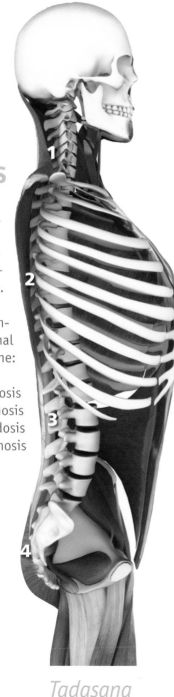

We determine the spinal curves by viewing them from the side. Kyphosis is a convex curve and lordosis is a concave curve.

This illustration demonstrates the four normal curves in the spine:

1) cervical lordosis
2) thoracic kyphosis
3) lumbar lordosis
4) sacral kyphosis

Tadasana

Add side planks

Scoliosis — lateral deviation / large misalignment

Scoliosis is a lateral deviation and rotational deformity of the spine. The most common form of scoliosis is called "idiopathic," meaning without an identifiable cause. Other forms include congenital and neuromuscular scoliosis. Studies have suggested that idiopathic scoliosis is related to hormonal factors, including the level of melatonin produced. This form of scoliosis also has a hereditary component.

When the magnitude of the scoliotic curve progresses beyond 20 degrees, there is a risk of continued progression after skeletal maturity. Very large scoliotic curves can impact respiration by restricting the ribcage.

Scoliosis also affects the pelvic and shoulder girdles, as illustrated here. For example, tilting the pelvic girdle creates a perception of limb length discrepancy (one leg shorter than the other). Similarly, one arm may appear shorter than the other.

Scoliosis affects the bone, cartilage, and muscles of the spine. Muscles on the concave side of a curve become chronically shortened when compared with those on the convex side. Yoga postures aid to counteract this process by stretching the shortened muscles.

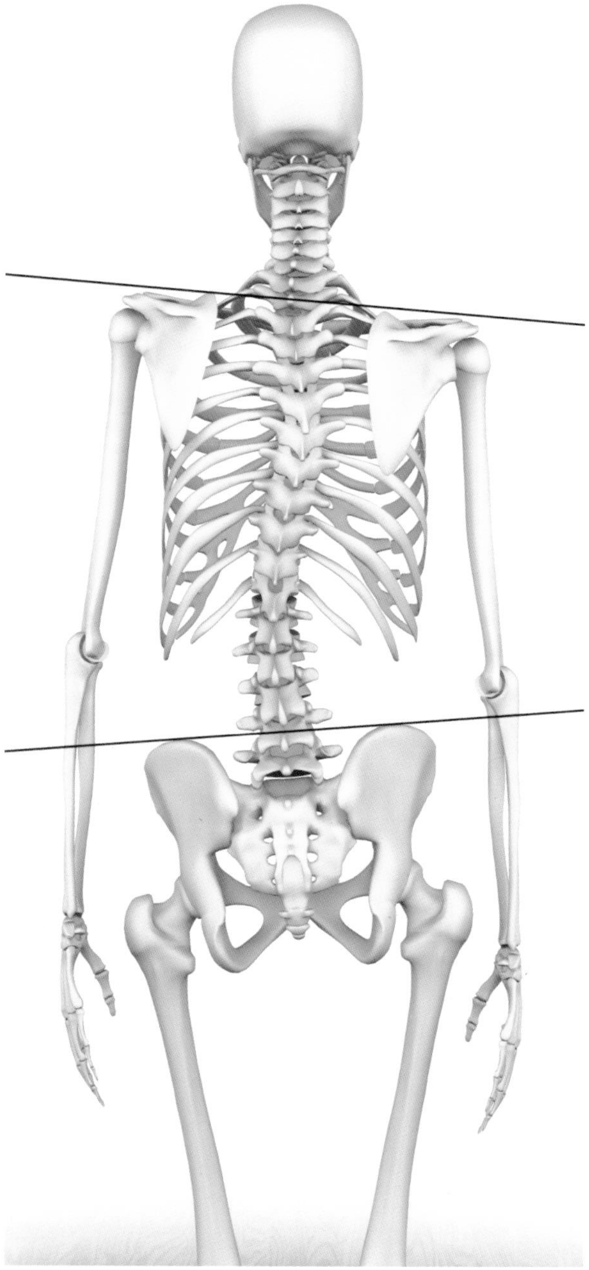

scoliosis

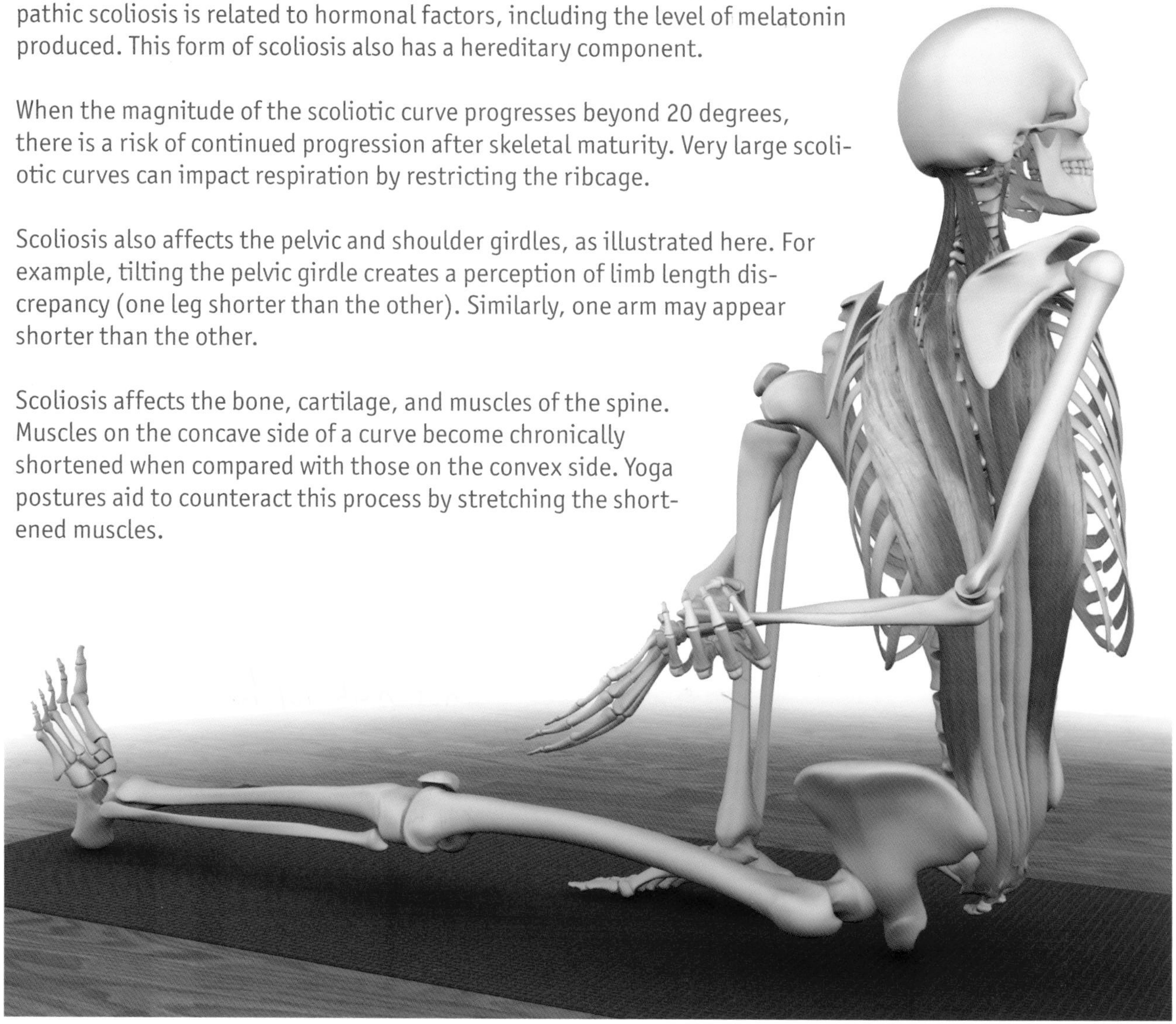

Marichyasana

Yoga as Therapy

These images of a twist, back bend, and forward bend demonstrate how Yoga postures contract and stretch the back muscles. This lengthens chronically shortened muscles on the concave side of the scoliotic curve while strengthening them on the convex side. This assists in balancing perceived discrepancies in limb length and may also improve nerve conduction.

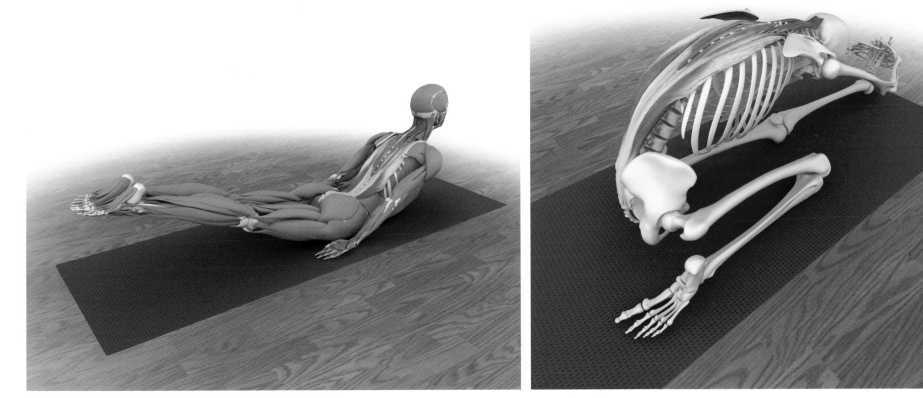

Salabhasana

Trianga Mukhaikapada Paschimottanasana

Joints

As with the bones, the shape of the joints reflects their function (and their function reflects their shape). Joints come in a spectrum of shapes, depending on the mobility or stability they require. For example, the hip joint is a ball and socket, while the knee joint is a hinge. A ball and socket hip joint confers the greatest mobility in all planes and is useful for activities, such as changing direction while walking and running (or reaching in various directions to grasp objects, as with the shoulder). A hinge joint, such as the knee, provides greater stability and is useful for propelling the body forward (or drawing an object toward the body, as with the elbow).

Other joints, such as the intervertebral joints between the vertebrae, allow for limited mobility between individual vertebrae but great stability to protect the spinal cord. Mobility of the spinal column comes from combining the limited movement of individual intervertebral joints as a whole.

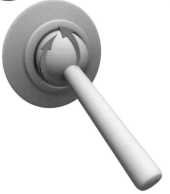

Circumduction

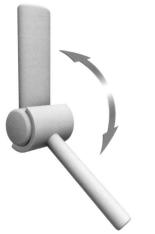

ball and socket

hinge

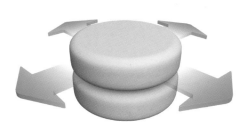

compressive

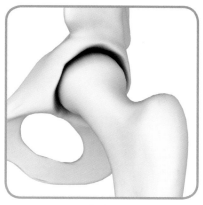

hip

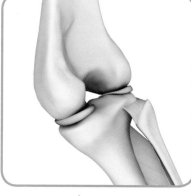

knee

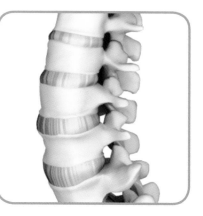

lumbar spine

Articular Structure

The joint capsule is connective tissue sheathing that surrounds and seals synovial joints. It is susceptible to stretch injury when executing extreme movements in Yoga postures.

Synovial tissue lines the inside of the joint capsule. This tissue produces synovial fluid, a viscous lubricant for the joint surface that decreases friction during joint movement. Synovial fluid circulates throughout the joint, transporting nutrients to the articular cartilage and removing debris from the joint space. The various contortions resulting from Yoga postures aid flexion and expansion of the joint capsule, stimulating circulation of synovial fluid.

Articular cartilage covers the joint surfaces, allowing smooth gliding of one bone over the other. In fact, articular cartilage is one of the smoothest surfaces known to humankind. Applying excessive pressure to this fragile cartilage can injure it, ultimately resulting in arthritis.

The meniscus deepens the articular surface and broadens the contact area of the joint. This aids to stabilize the joint and distributes the force of gravity and muscular contraction over a greater surface area. The meniscus is composed of fibrocartilage, giving it a flexible rubbery consistency.

hip articular cartilage

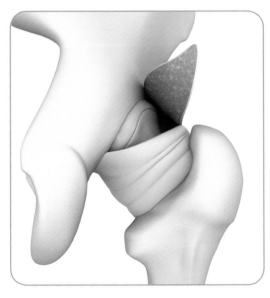

hip joint capsule with synovium (posterior view)

knee with menisci

23

Fundamentals
Joint Reaction Forces

Every action has an equal and opposite reaction. Muscular contraction and gravity create opposing forces across the joint surfaces, known as joint reaction forces. It is important to spread these forces over the greatest possible joint surface area.

Joint congruency refers to the fit of a joint's articular surfaces. A joint is congruent when its surfaces fit together perfectly. Movement out of congruency focuses stress on a small surface area. A large force focused on a small area of articular cartilage can injure it, eventually causing degenerative changes.

Some Yoga postures have the capacity to sublux or take a joint into an incongruent position. Avoid this by using the joints with a greater range of motion while protecting those joints with limited range of motion.

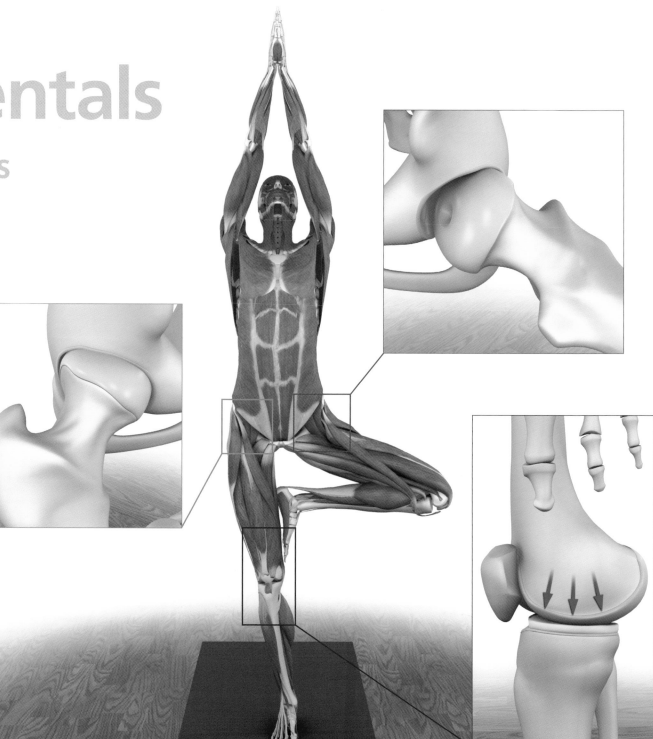

Joint Reaction Forces—Applied

For example, the ball and socket joint of the hip has greater range of motion than the hinge joint of the knee. Lotus posture (or Padmasana) requires a large amount of external rotation of the hip joint to bring the foot into position on the opposite leg. Obtaining this external rotation from the knee joint creates incongruency because the knee is a hinge joint with limited capacity to rotate. This incongruency can result in the abnormal distribution of joint reaction forces, injuring the intra-articular structures of the knee. Therefore it is essential to first obtain full range of motion of the ball and socket hip joint to protect the hinge knee joint (see arrows).

Ardha Padmasana

Ligaments

Hold bones in place

no blood flow

Ligaments are fibrous connective tissue structures that link one bone to another at the joint. They serve to stabilize the joint, while at the same time allowing mobility. Ligaments vary in size and shape according to their function. For example, the cruciate ligaments of the knee are short, stout structures that assist in maintaining the knee as a hinge. The sacroiliac ligaments are dense, broad, and thick structures that limit movement of the sacroiliac joint. The shoulder ligaments are thin band-like structures that are confluent with the shoulder capsule, allowing for great range of motion.

Ligaments are non-contractile, but they actively participate in movement because they have sensory nerves that transmit information about joint position to the spinal cord and brain.

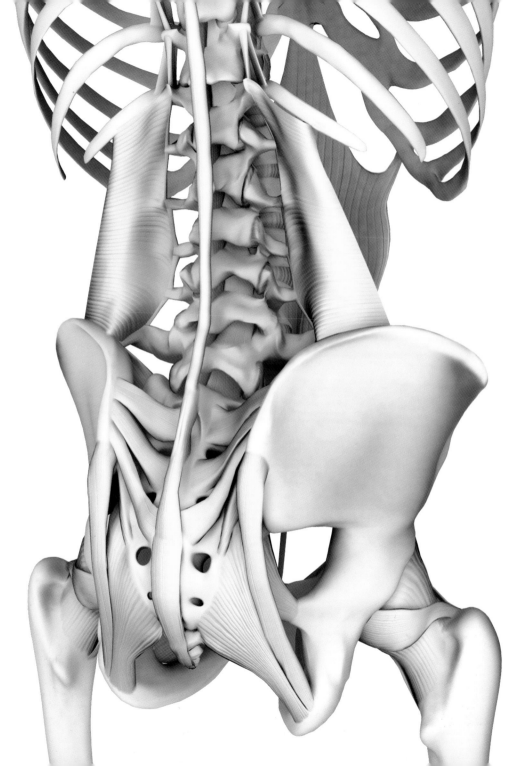

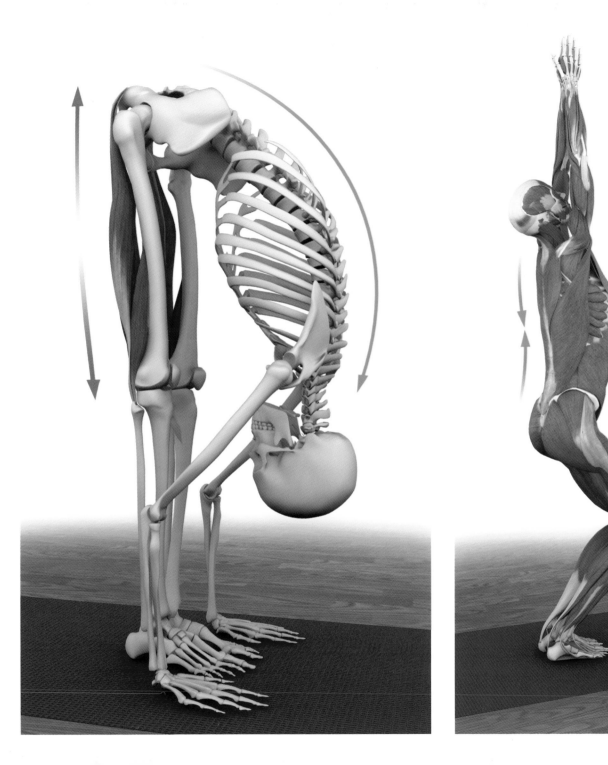

Ligamentotaxis

Ligamentotaxis refers to the pull of ligaments on the bones to which they are attached. This concept is used by physicians to pull broken bones back into place and set them. It can also be used during Yoga practice as illustrated here in the forward bend, Uttanasana. Here the weight of the upper body is transmitted to the pelvis via the ligaments of the back. This pulls the pelvis forward and lifts the ischial tuberosities, passively stretching the hamstrings. Similarly, ligaments have some capacity for elastic recoil. This recoil can be combined with the momentum of the body as it raises from postures such as back bends.

27

Pelvic and Hip Ligaments

The form of the pelvic and hip ligaments reflects their function. The pelvic ligaments are thick and strong in support of the weight bearing function of these joints. The hip ligaments are shaped to stabilize the hip while allowing movement for walking and running.

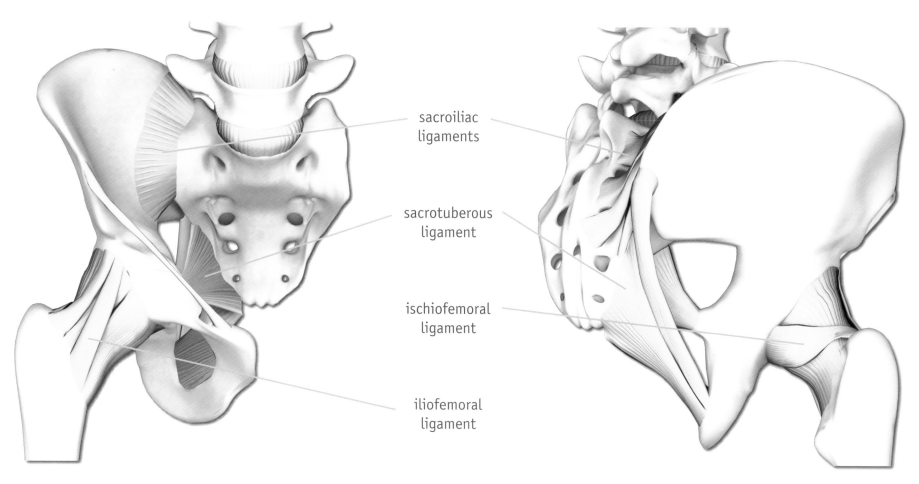

sacroiliac
ligaments

sacrotuberous
ligament

ischiofemoral
ligament

iliofemoral
ligament

Pelvis and Hip (anterior)

Pelvis and Hip (posterior)

Iliofemoral Ligaments

The iliofemoral ligament is part of the hip joint that works to stabilize the hip. This ligament becomes taut when the femur extends and externally rotates. It relaxes when the femur flexes and internally rotates. Tightness in this ligament limits extension of the hip in lunging poses and forward splits. This limitation is overcome by tilting the pelvis forward and internally rotating the femur.

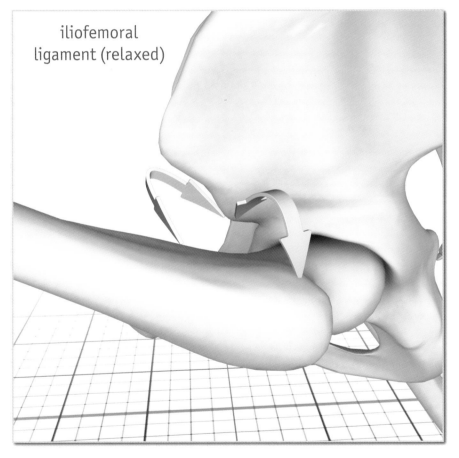

iliofemoral
ligament (relaxed)

Hip Joint (flexed, internally rotated)

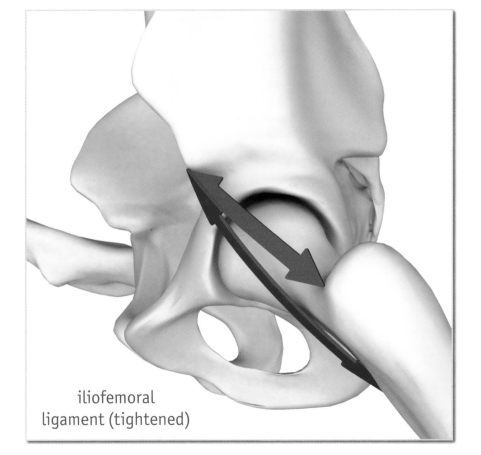

iliofemoral
ligament (tightened)

Hip Joint (extended, externally rotated)

Shoulder and Elbow Ligaments

Elbow (posterior)

The collateral ligaments of the elbow limit side-to-side motion and maintain the joint as a hinge. The interosseous membrane stabilizes the bones of the forearm.

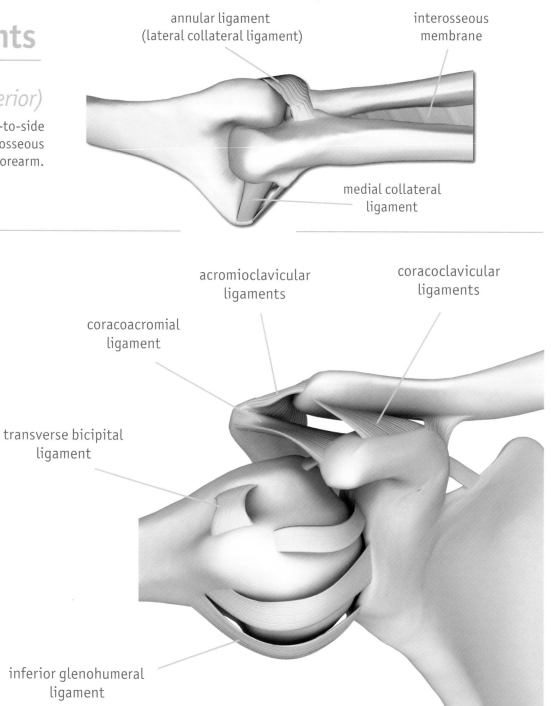

annular ligament
(lateral collateral ligament)

interosseous membrane

medial collateral ligament

acromioclavicular ligaments

coracoclavicular ligaments

coracoacromial ligament

transverse bicipital ligament

inferior glenohumeral ligament

Shoulder

Unlike the thick ligaments of the hip, the glenohumeral ligaments of the shoulder are thin structures. Their design allows greater mobility of the joint.

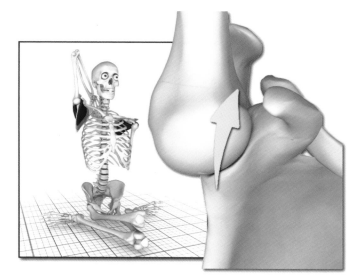

The inferior glenohumeral ligament is the most important of the three glenohumeral ligaments. This ligament tightens when the humerus abducts and externally rotates.

The Muscular Stabilizers of the Shoulder

The shape of the bones and thick ligaments stabilize the hip. Muscles stabilize the shoulder. The primary shoulder stabilizer is the rotator cuff; the secondary stabilizers are the triceps and biceps. Yoga postures, such as arm balances and inversions, strengthen these muscles, balancing stability and mobility in the joint.

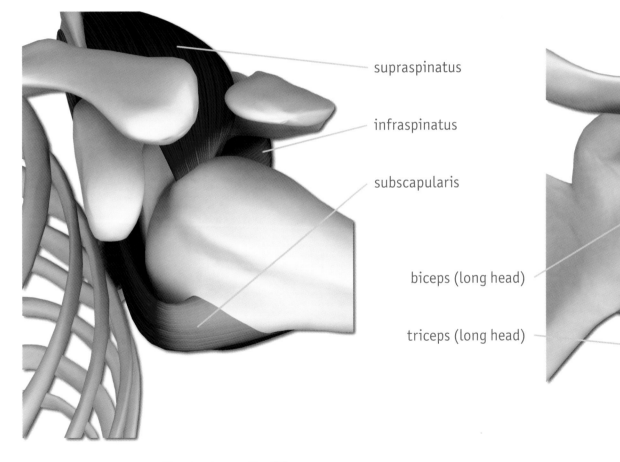

supraspinatus

infraspinatus

subscapularis

biceps (long head)

triceps (long head)

*Rotator Cuff
(stabilizing shoulder joint)*

*Biceps and Triceps
(stabilizing shoulder joint)*

Spine Ligaments

The vertebral unit is comprised of two adjacent vertebral bodies and the intervertebral disc. Movement between the vertebrae is possible in several planes (including small amounts of rotation, flexion, and extension). The combination of motion across multiple vertebral units culminates in spinal movement.

LUMBOSACRAL SPINE

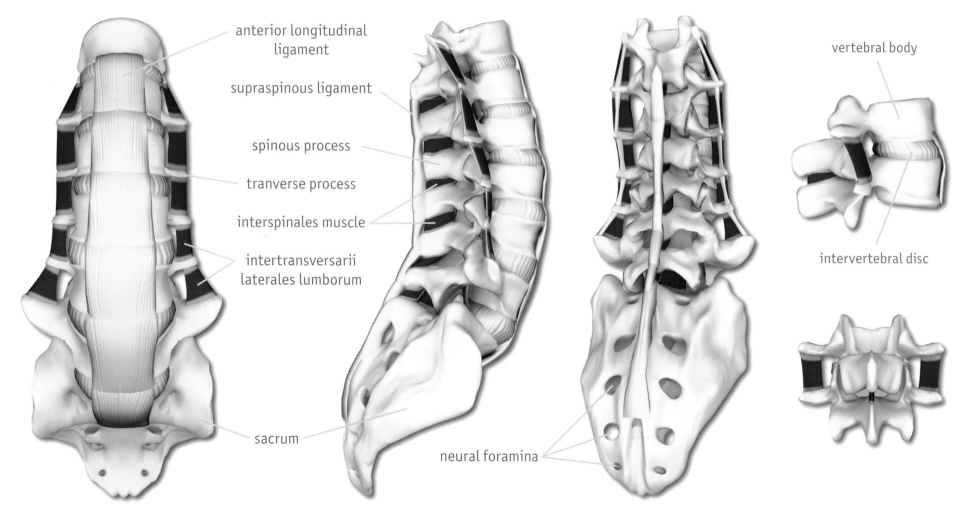

anterior longitudinal ligament

supraspinous ligament

spinous process

tranverse process

interspinales muscle

intertransversarii laterales lumborum

sacrum

neural foramina

vertebral body

intervertebral disc

Trunk Ligaments

Ligaments attach bone to bone and also serve as attachments for certain muscles. Below are three such ligaments that connect the upper body and trunk with the lower body.

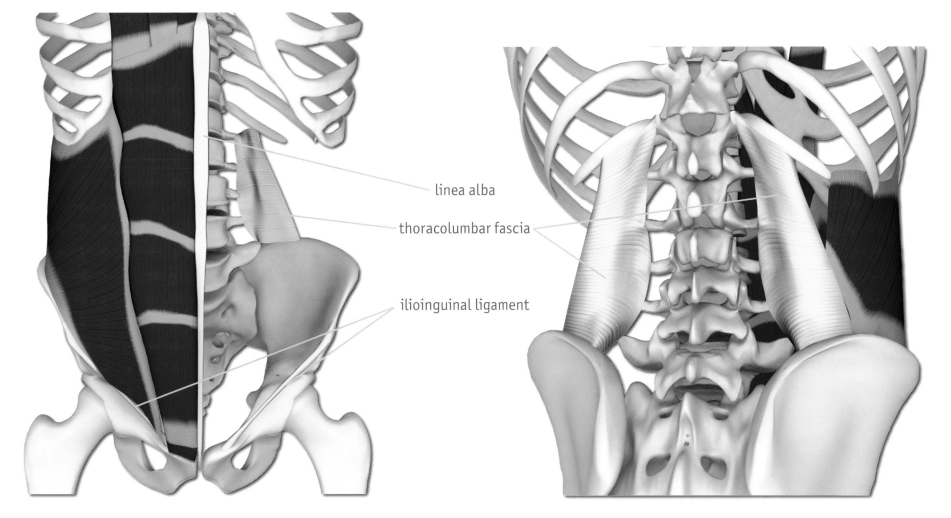

linea alba

thoracolumbar fascia

ilioinguinal ligament

Trunk (anterior)

Trunk (posterior)

Knee Ligaments

The patellar tendon connects the quadriceps muscle to the tibia for extension of the knee. The collateral ligaments limit side-to-side motion of the knee and maintain its function as a hinge joint. The anterior and posterior cruciate ligaments limit anterior and posterior translation of the tibia on the femur, respectively. The menisci deepen and stabilize the knee joint. The interosseous membrane stabilizes the bones of the lower leg.

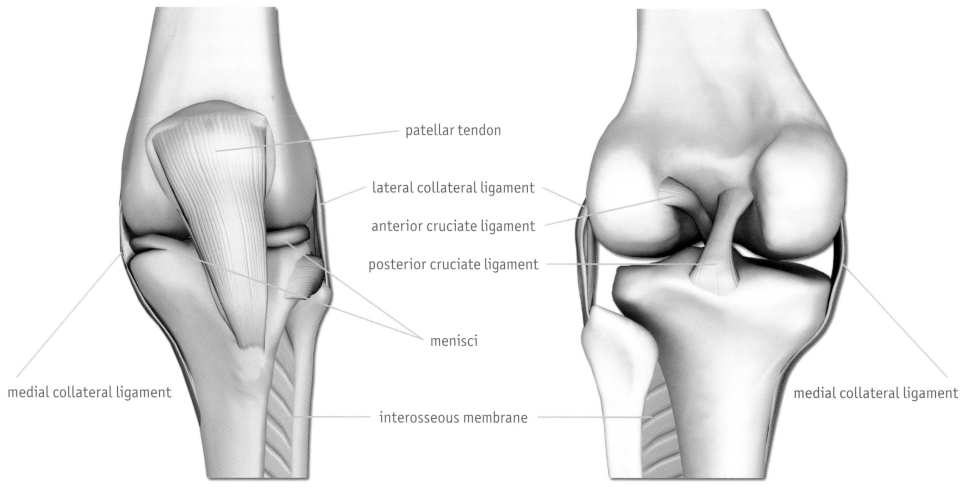

patellar tendon

lateral collateral ligament

anterior cruciate ligament

posterior cruciate ligament

menisci

medial collateral ligament

interosseous membrane

medial collateral ligament

Knee (anterior)

Knee (posterior with menisci removed)

Muscles and Tendons

Muscles

Movements are determined by the varying forces acting across the joints. These forces are produced by the muscles, and their effects on body position are determined by the muscles' shape, origin (the attachment of the muscle to a bone at the more fixed or proximal end), and insertion (the attachment of the muscle to a bone at the end toward the part to be moved, or the more distal end).

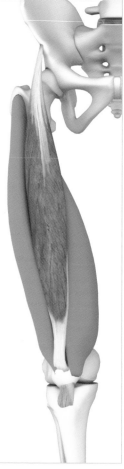

The origin of the rectus femoris is the anterior superior iliac spine. The insertion is the patella.

Origin
Proximal attachment of the muscle to a bone.

Insertion
Distal attachment of the muscle to a bone.

Agonist, or Prime Mover
The muscle that contracts to produce a certain action about a joint. For example, the hamstrings are agonists when you flex your knee.

Antagonist
A muscle that relaxes while the agonist contracts. The antagonist produces the opposite action about a joint. For example, the quadriceps (at the front of the thigh) are the antagonists to the hamstrings when you flex your knee. When you extend your knee, the quadriceps are the agonists and the hamstrings are the antagonists.

Synergist
A muscle that assists and fine-tunes the action of the agonist and which can be used to produce the same action, although generally not as efficiently.

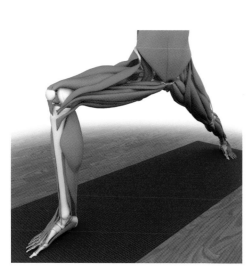

The synergists of the psoas assist in flexing the hip.

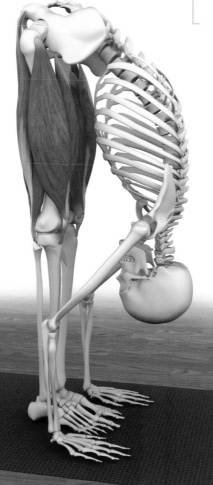

The quadriceps are the agonists that contract to extend the knees. The hamstrings are the antagonists stretched by this action.

Muscles and Tendons

Tendons attach muscles to bones, transmitting the forces produced by the muscles, moving joints. Tendons also have sensory nerves that communicate information about muscle tension and joint position to the brain.
Tendons and ligaments have limited capacity to stretch and do not contract. Practicing Yoga improves tendon and ligament flexibility, especially when performed in a heated room. Practitioners should not stretch tendons or ligaments beyond their normal length, as this can cause injury.

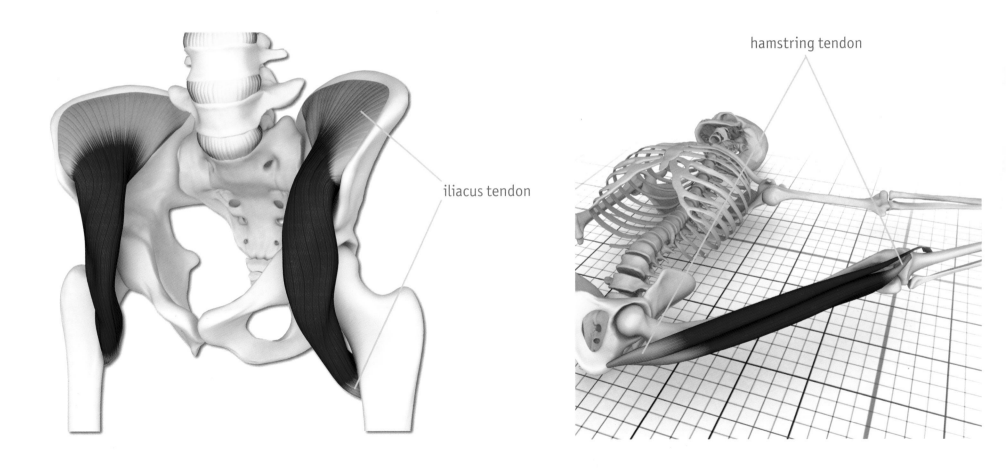

iliacus tendon

hamstring tendon

Muscle Shapes

Muscles come in a variety of shapes, reflecting their specific function. These different shapes provide for maximal mechanical efficiency during movement of the skeleton. Similarly, muscles may curve over the bones to provide a "half-pulley" effect which multiplies the force of contraction. Some of the various muscle shapes include the following:

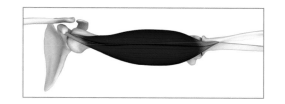

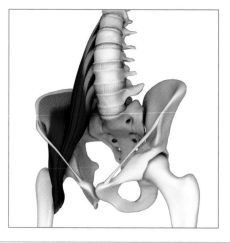

biceps brachialis
two-headed fusiform

iliopsoas
multiheaded convergent
(with half-pulley)

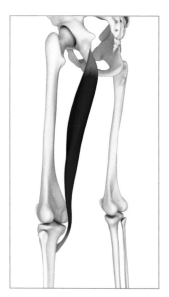

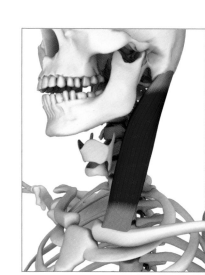

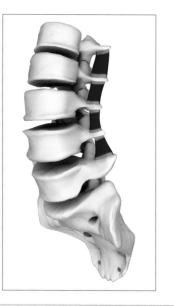

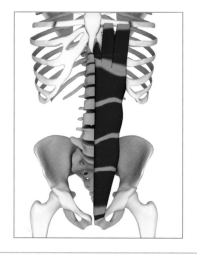

semitendinosus
one-headed fusiform

sternocleidomastoid
strap

intertransversarii laterales
lumborum - short square

latissimus dorsi
triangular convergent

rectus abdominis
flat aponeurotic

Monoarticular and Polyarticular Muscles

Muscles are also defined by the number of joints that they cross from their origin to their insertion. Monoarticular muscles cross only one joint, while polyarticular muscles cross more than one joint.

When monoarticular muscles contract, they primarily move only one joint. When polyarticular muscles contract, they can move multiple joints.

For example, in the one-legged Vrksasana, the iliacus and gluteus medius represent monoarticular muscles because they originate on the ilium and attach to the proximal femur, crossing (and moving) only the hip joint. Here the iliacus and gluteus medius serve to stabilize the hip joint in the standing leg. The quadratus lumborum, psoas, rectus femoris, and sartorius represent polyarticular muscles because they all cross (and move) multiple joints. Here these muscles contribute to flexing, abducting, and externally rotating the non-standing leg.

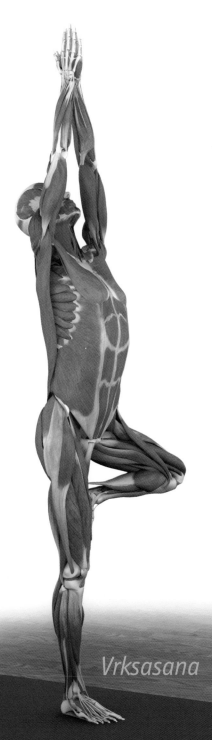

Vrksasana

monoarticular

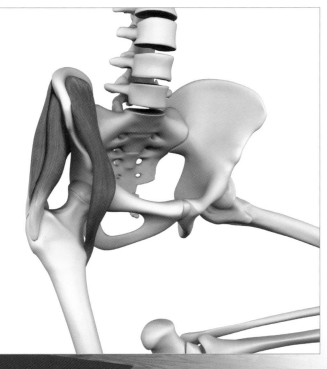

polyarticular

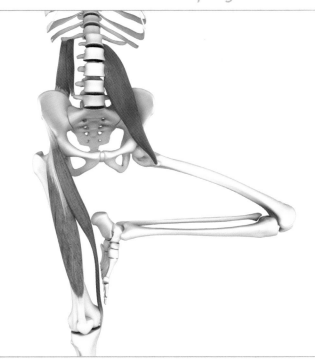

39

Muscle Structure and Function

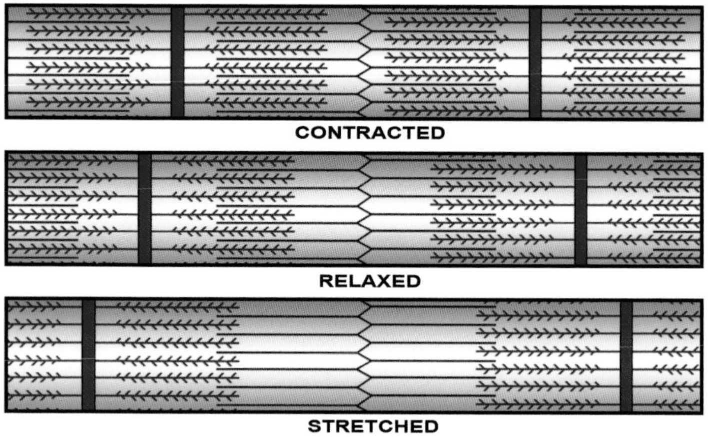

CONTRACTED

RELAXED

STRETCHED

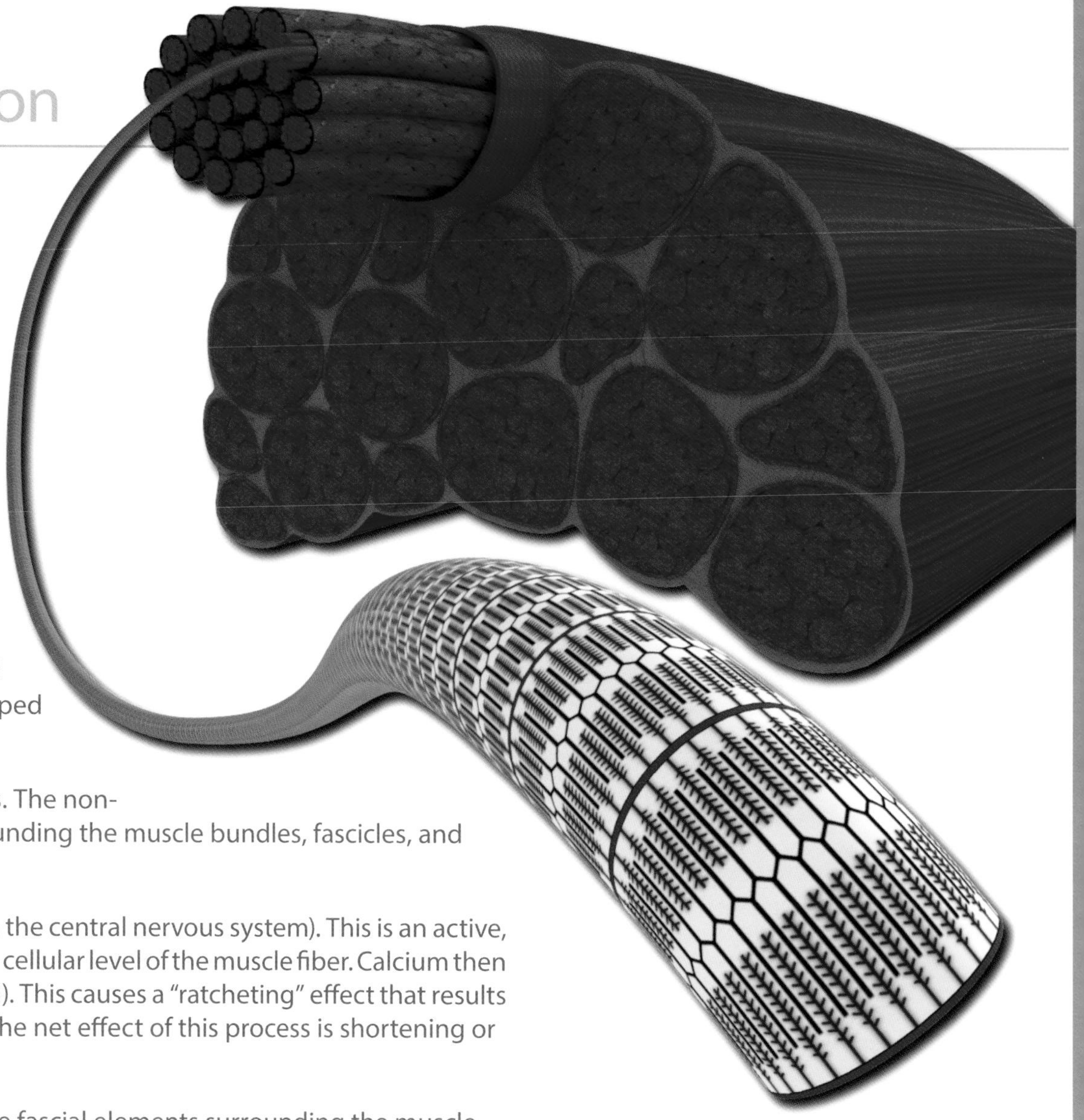

Muscle fibers are the functional contractile units of each skeletal muscle. Fibers are grouped into fascicles which, in turn, are grouped into bundles, thus forming the individual skeletal muscles.

Skeletal muscles are also composed of non-contractile elements. The non-contractile elements include the connective tissue sheath surrounding the muscle bundles, fascicles, and individual fibers, as well as the myotendon junction.

Muscle fibers contract in response to efferent nerve stimuli (from the central nervous system). This is an active, energy-dependent process involving the release of calcium at the cellular level of the muscle fiber. Calcium then forms cross-bridging between the myofilaments (of the myofibril). This causes a "ratcheting" effect that results in the shortening or contraction of the individual muscle fiber. The net effect of this process is shortening or contraction of the entire muscle.

The force of this contraction is transmitted to the non-contractile fascial elements surrounding the muscle. These fascial elements then transmit this force to the myotendon junction and on to the bones, moving the joint.

Muscles exist in either a contracted, relaxed, or stretched state. This is illustrated above in the inset showing the cross-bridging of myofilaments.

Types of Muscle Contraction

There are three types of muscle contraction:

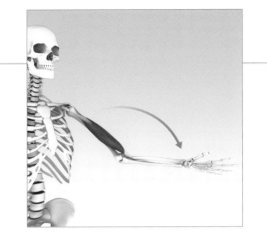

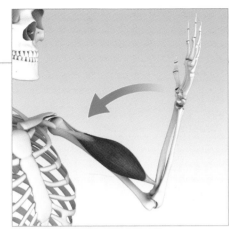

Concentric (Isotonic) Contraction:

The muscle shortens while maintaining constant tension through a range of motion.

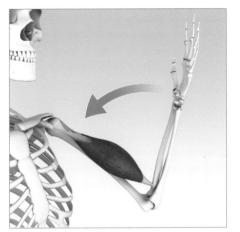

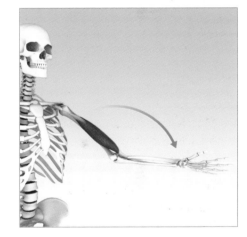

Eccentric Contraction:

The muscle contracts while lengthening.

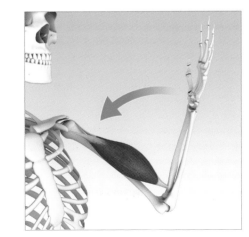

Isometric Contraction:

The muscle generates tension but does not shorten, and the bones do not move.

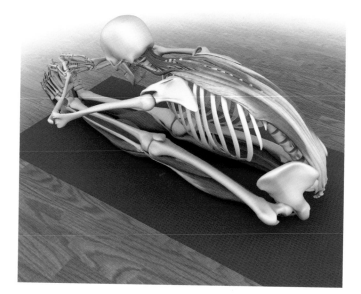

Stretching Muscles

Static Stretching

Static stretching is the most common technique used in Hatha Yoga. There are two categories of static stretching. The first is active static stretching. This involves contracting antagonist muscles to stretch a target muscle. Contracting the quadriceps, iliopsoas, and biceps during the forward bend Paschimottanasana is a form of active static stretching of the hamstrings. Contracting antagonist muscles in active static stretching results in a phenomenon called "reciprocal inhibition." During reciprocal inhibition, the central nervous system signals the target muscle to relax.

Passive static stretching occurs when we relax into a stretch, using only the force of body weight (or an externally applied weight) to stretch muscles. The restorative pose Suported Setu Bandha Sarvangasana is an example of passive static stretching of the iliopsoas muscle.

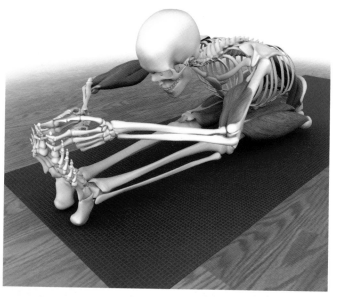

active static stretching

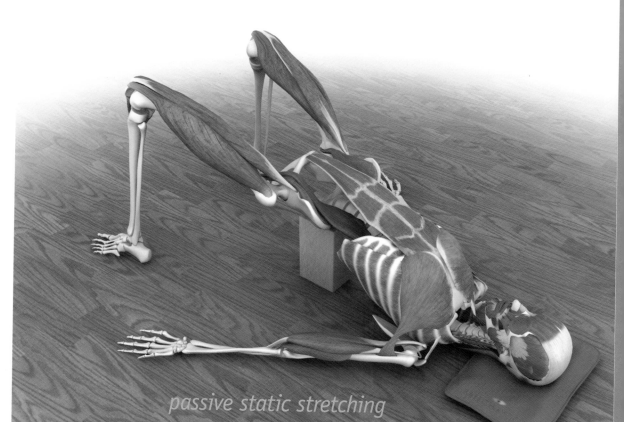

passive static stretching

Facilitated Stretching

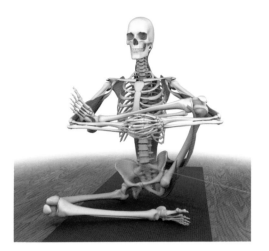

Yoga practitioners use facilitated stretching to deepen their postures. This type of stretching involves contracting the muscle being stretched during an active static stretch. This action triggers a reflex arc involving the Golgi tendon organ, resulting in a profound relaxation of the target muscle when the contraction period ends. This is also known as proprioceptive neuromuscular facilitation (PNF). It is extremely important to consider the joint reaction forces when using facilitated stretches, since the force the muscle generates is transmitted to the joints. As a general rule, gently contract the stretched muscle to avoid excessive joint reaction forces. These images demonstrate facilitated stretching of the gluteus medius, gluteus maximus, and tensor fascia lata.

Dynamic Stretching

Yoga practitioners use dynamic stretching during a Vinyasa style of practice. This type of stretching involves repetitive movement of the body into increasingly deeper stretches. Performing dynamic stretching in the morning "resets" the resting muscle length for the day.

(Scientific Keys, Volume II, covers the physiology of stretching in detail).

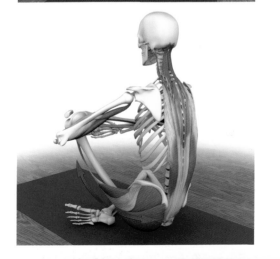

Movement

Movement Definitions

Motion of the musculoskeletal system necessarily involves multiple joints, forces applied in many directions, and movement in many planes. A convention exists to describe the basic movements of the musculoskeletal system that can be useful in analyzing the form and function of the Asanas.

The six basic movements of the body take place in three planes.

Coronal plane: Divides the body into front and back. Movements along this plane are called adduction and abduction. Adduction moves the extremity toward the midline, abduction moves the extremity away from the midline.

Sagittal plane: Divides the body into right and left. Movements along this plane are called flexion and extension. Flexion usually moves the extremity forward, except at the knee, where it moves backward. Extension moves the extremity backward.

Transverse plane: Divides the body into upper and lower halves. Movement along this plane is called rotation. Rotation is further classified as medial rotation (toward the midline) or lateral rotation (away from the midline). Medial and lateral rotation are also referred to as internal and external rotation, respectively.

All movements of the body are composed of varying contributions of these six elemental movements.

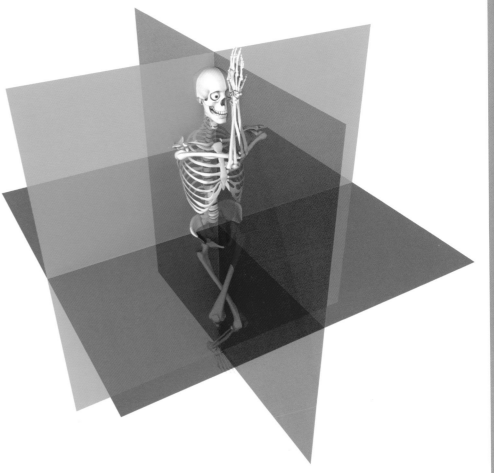

Pose with Movements

The form of each Asana reflects its function and vice versa. Here we use Virabhadrasana II to analyze the positions of the body in a Yoga posture. You can combine this analysis with knowledge of the muscle actions to optimize the function of your poses.

1. The front knee flexes.

2. The front hip flexes.

3. The back hip extends.

4. The back foot rotates internally.

5. The torso extends.

6. The arms abduct.

7. The forearms rotate internally.

8. The neck and head rotate.

Virabhadrasana II

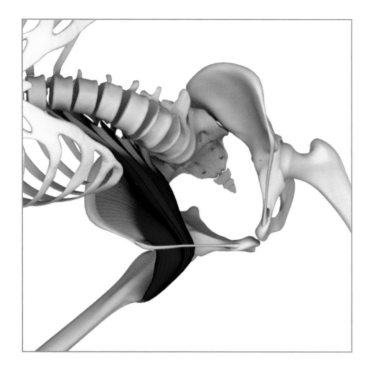

Complex Movements

In reality, and especially in Yoga postures, movement can rarely be described in simple terms. Complex movements involve many joints moving in various ways. Complex movements are also described in terms of other characteristics, including coupling of joints and open- and closed-chain movements.

Coupling of Joints

Movement of adjacent joints in different planes is called coupled movement. For example, in the side bend of Utthita Trikonasana, the vertebral column undergoes a complex series of coupled movements, including rotation, flexion, and extension at various levels. Similarly, in the same pose, the position of the hip joint of the forward leg combines flexion of the femur (thigh bone) at the hip joint and forward tilt of the pelvis.

Open- and Closed-Chain Movements

1) Open chain: Movements in which the distal end moves freely (for example, the deltoid abducting the upper arms in Virabhadrasana II).

2) Closed chain: Movements in which the distal end (the insertion) of the moving limb or body segment are fixed (for example, the iliopsoas lowering the pelvis in Virabhadrasana II).

Open-chain movements teach balance and awareness of the body in space. Closed-chain movements strengthen the core muscles.

Part One

Pelvic Girdle & Thighs

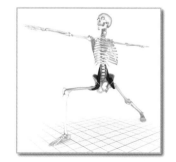 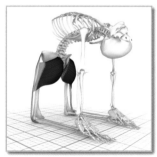 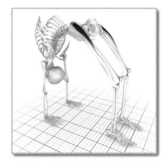 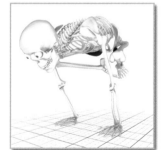 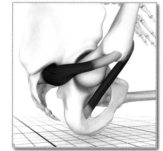 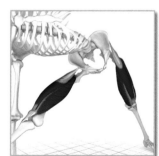

External Rotators of the Hip

1 piriformis

2 superior gamellus

3 obturator internus

4 inferior gamellus

5 quadratus femoris

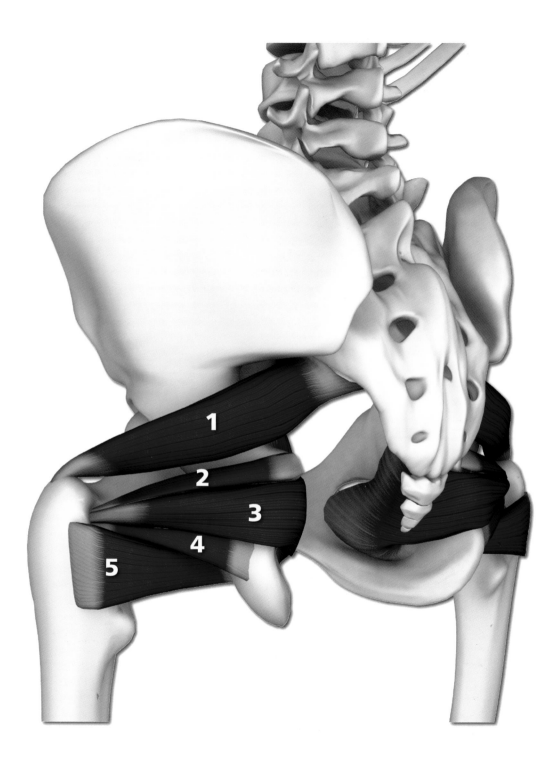

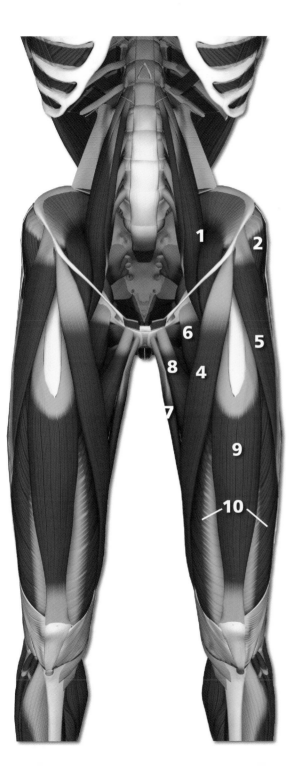

1	iliopsoas
2	gluteus medius
3	gluteus maximus
4	sartorius
5	tensor fascia lata
6	pectineus
7	gracilis
8	adductor longus
9	rectus femoris
10	quadriceps
11	biceps femoris
12	semitendinosus
13	semimembranosus
14	gastrocnemius

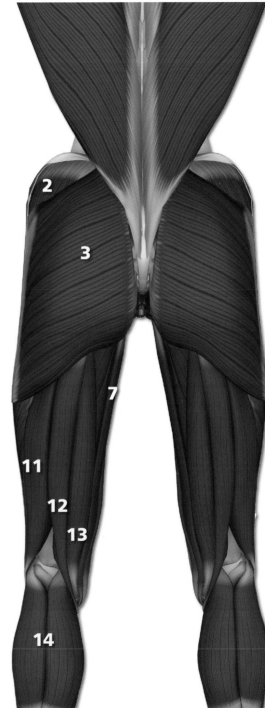

Movement: Hip

The following examples illustrate the elemental movements of the hip and pelvis. Look closely to appreciate the "coupling" of the movements of the hip joint and pelvis.

Flexion
Utthita Hasta Padangusthasana

Extension
Vrishchikasana

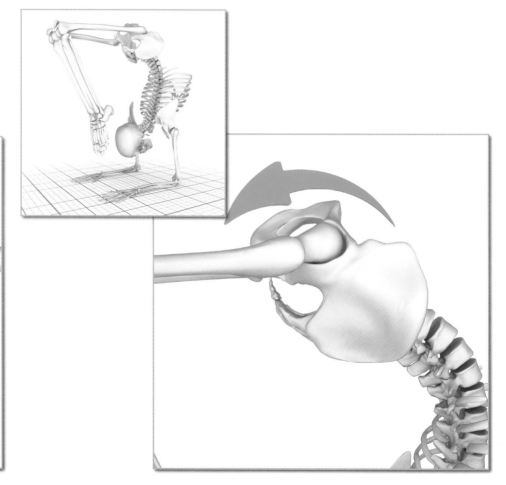

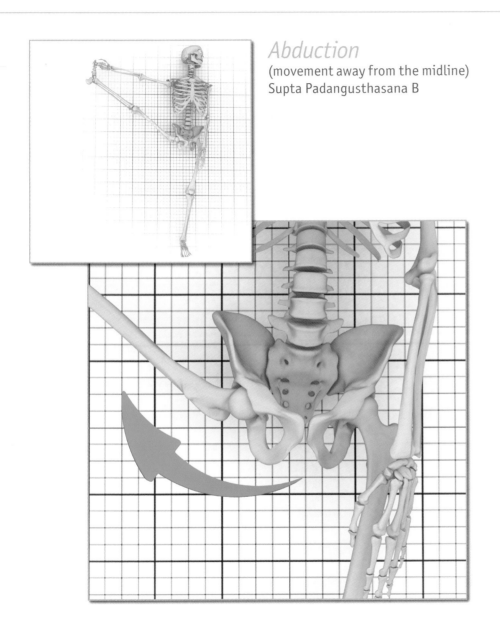

Abduction
(movement away from the midline)
Supta Padangusthasana B

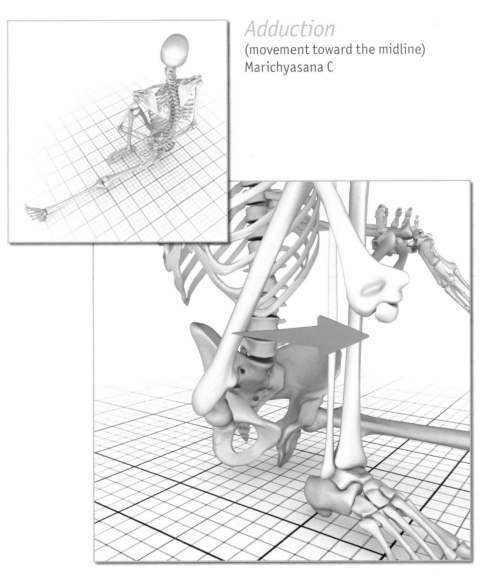

Adduction
(movement toward the midline)
Marichyasana C

Movement: Hip

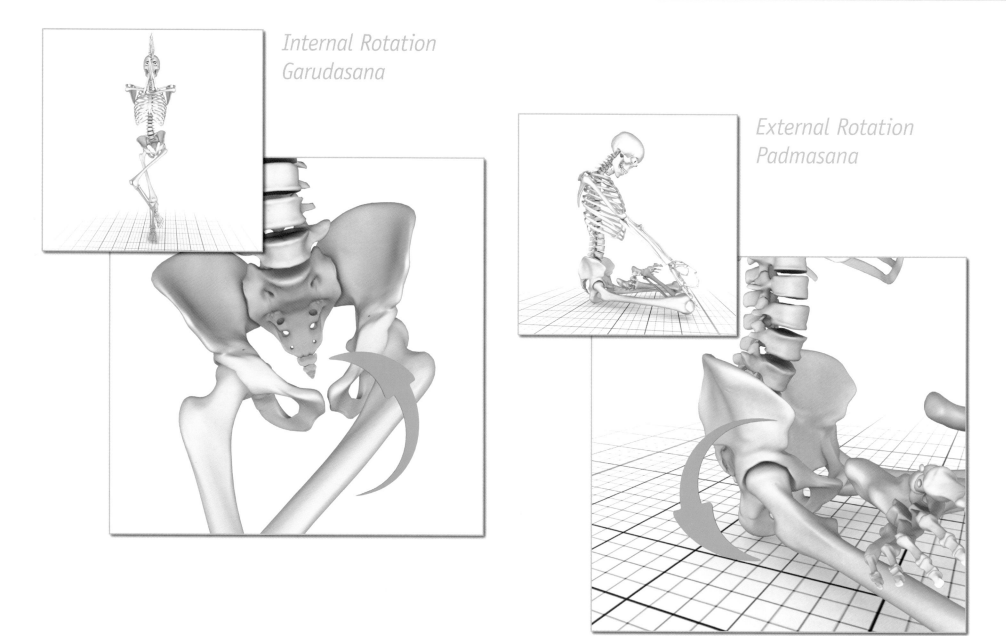

Internal Rotation
Garudasana

External Rotation
Padmasana

Movement: Pelvis

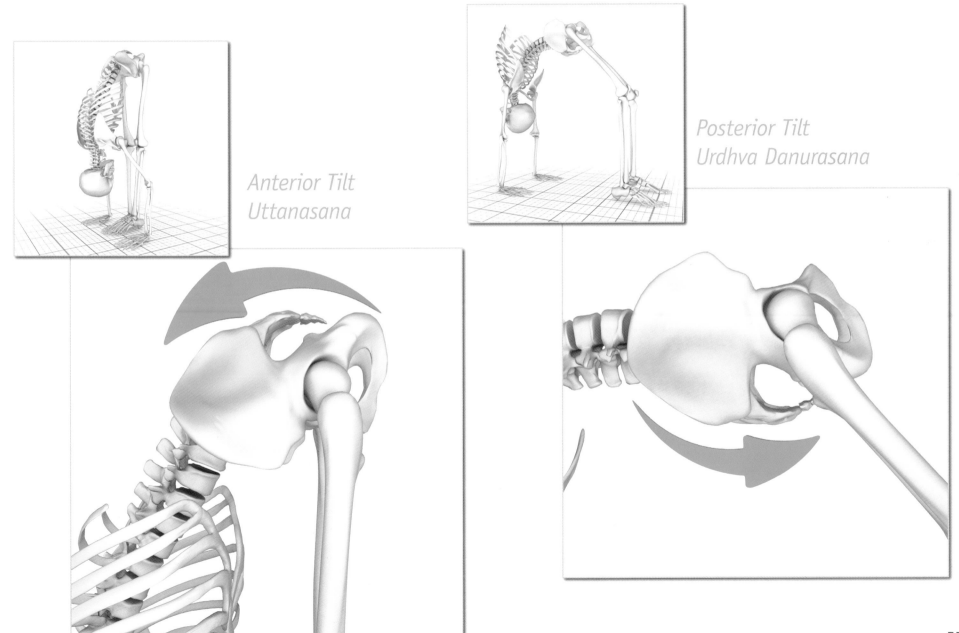

Anterior Tilt
Uttanasana

Posterior Tilt
Urdhva Danurasana

Movement: Pelvis

Rotation
Garudasana

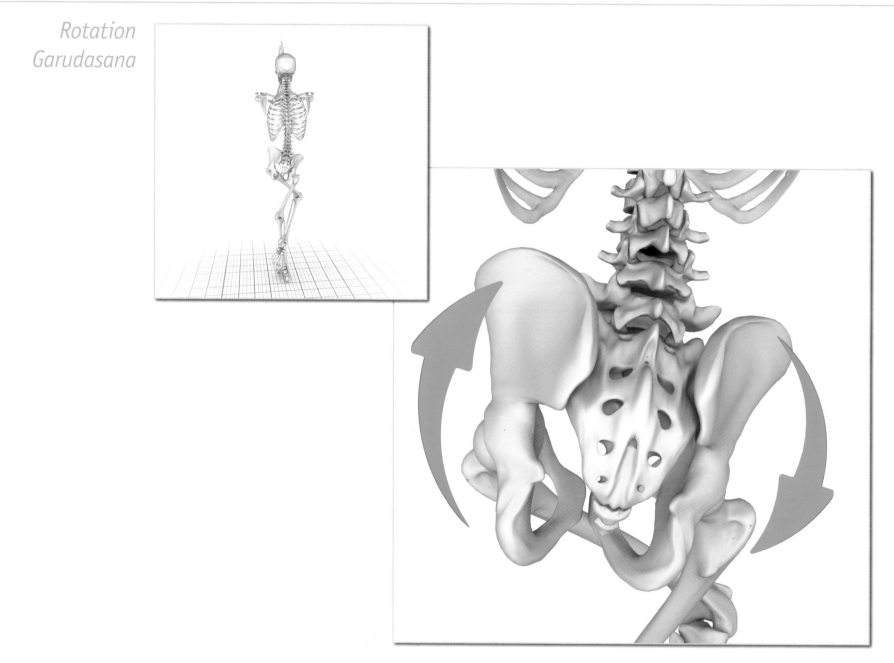

Chapter 1

Iliopsoas

Also known as the psoas muscle, the iliopsoas is actually a combination of two large muscles: the psoas major and the iliacus. The psoas major muscle originates in the lower back; the iliacus originates on the inside of the pelvis. Both muscles combine to form one tendon that attaches to the inside of the proximal femur bone.

psoas major

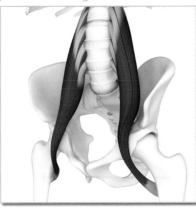

iliacus

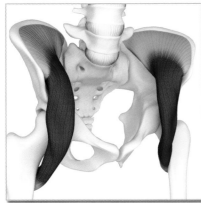

The iliopsoas is thus polyarticular. This means that it crosses over (and moves) more than one joint. The iliopsoas acts like a pulley as it curves over the front rim of the pelvis on its way to the femur. Like other pulley systems, this serves to multiply the force generated when the iliopsoas contracts. The iliopsoas thus moves the bones of the lower back, pelvis, and hip in a coupled fashion. This means that, when it contracts, a combination of movements across several joints is possible.

The iliopsoas first awakens during infancy when we are learning to sit up and then walk. Once awakened, the iliopsoas becomes constantly active in activities such as standing and walking. In spite of this constant use, our awareness of the iliopsoas quickly becomes unconscious. (Imagine if we had to think every time we took a step!)

Hatha Yoga can be used to reawaken our consciousness of this large and important muscle. Once you awaken the iliopsoas, contract or relax it to transform and deepen your Asanas.

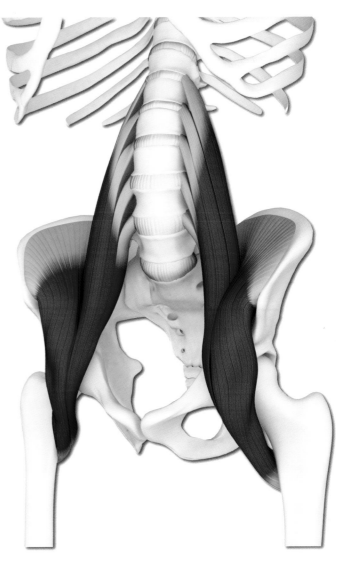

iliopsoas

Origin

1) Psoas major: Tranverse processes, discs, and bodies of lumbar vertebrae 1 through 5; body of the twelfth thoracic vertebra.

2) Iliacus: Upper two thirds of the inside surface of the iliac bone up to the inner lip of the iliac crest and anterior sacroiliac joint.

Innervation & Chakra Illuminated

Lumbar nerves 1,2,3,4.
Chakra: Second.

The second Chakra is illuminated by contracting and lengthening the iliopsoas muscle. This is due to stimulation of the various sensory nerves at its origin and insertion, within the muscle itself, and on the skin surrounding it.

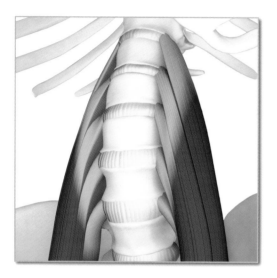

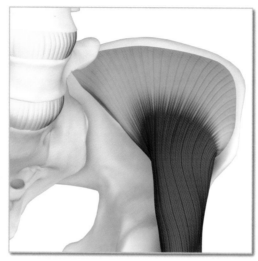

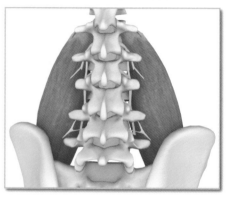

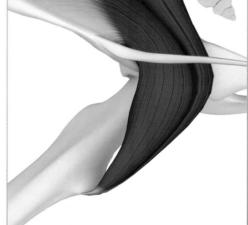

Insertion

Lesser trochanter (the smaller prominence or knob) of the proximal femur.

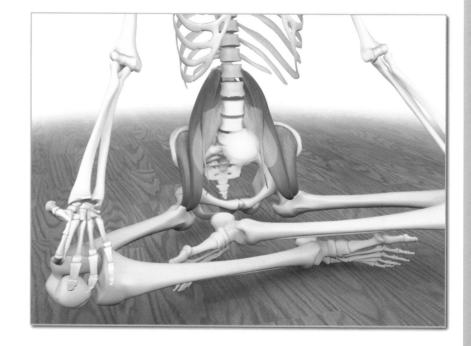

Iliopsoas (il-e-o-SO-us)

Antagonists

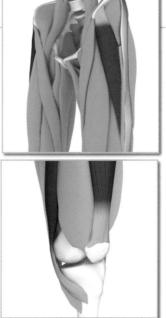

Tensor fascia lata: Assists the iliopsoas in fine-tuning hip flexion.

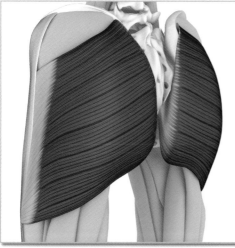

Gluteus maximus: Extends the hip and trunk, lengthening and stretching the iliopsoas, particularly in back bends.

Sartorius: Assists the iliopsoas in fine-tuning hip flexion and external rotation.

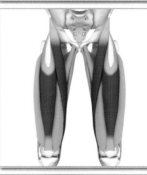

Rectus femoris: Assists the iliopsoas in fine-tuning hip flexion; it also assists the gluteus maximus in accentuating the stretch of the iliopsoas during back bending (by extending the knee).

Hamstrings: Extends the hip when initiating back bends; they can be used to draw the opposite leg iliopsoas into a deeper stretch in lunging postures.

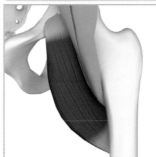

Pectineus: Assists the iliopsoas in fine-tuning hip flexion and provides an adduction component to stabilize the hip (also balances abduction action of sartorius).

59

Synergy

This illustration uses Virabhadrasana II to demonstrate the tensor fascia lata, sartorius, rectus femoris, and pectineus as synergists of the psoas. Similarly, the extended back hip demonstrates how the gluteus maximus and hamstrings act as antagonists to the psoas.

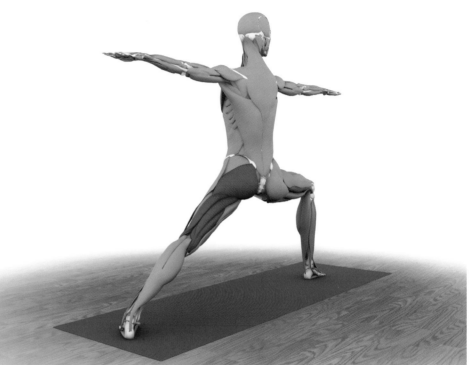

Virabhadrasana II

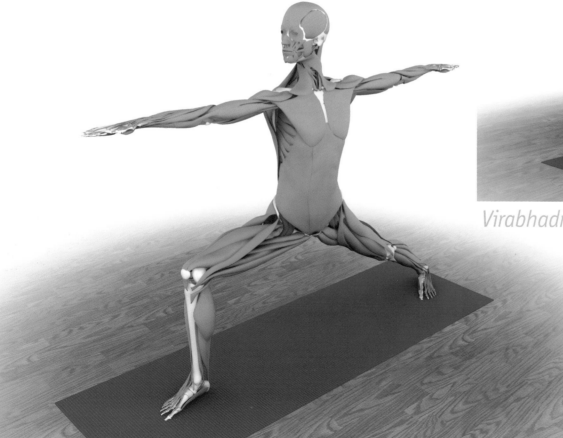

Synergy

This illustration uses Eka Pada Viparita Dandasana to demonstrate the gluteus maximus and hamstrings stretching the psoas and the synergists of the psoas in the planted leg. Similarly, the flexed hip of the leg in the air demonstrates the tensor fascia lata, sartorius, rectus femoris, and pectineus as synergists of the psoas.

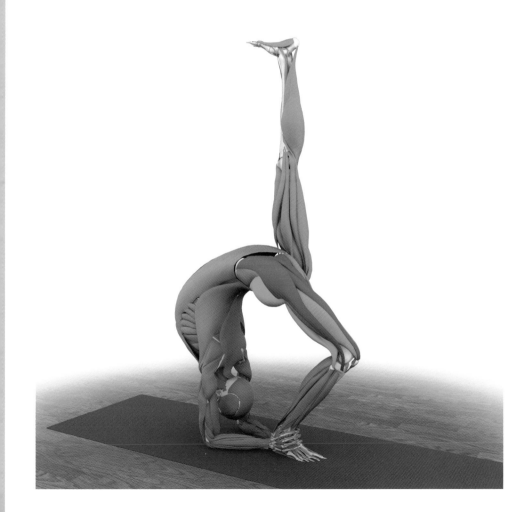

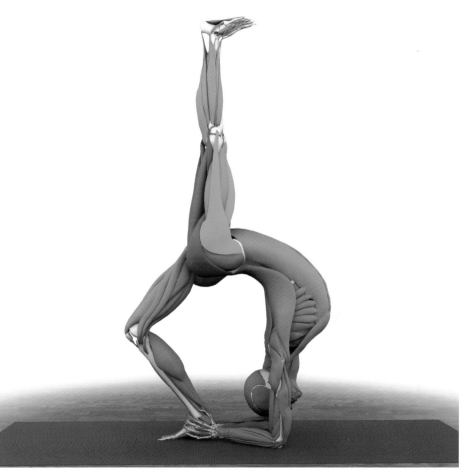

Eka Pada Viparita Dandasana

Iliopsoas (il-e-o-SO-us)

Action

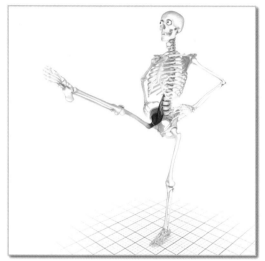

Open Chain
(Origin fixed, insertion moving):

Flexes and laterally rotates the femur at the hip, e.g., Utthita Hasta Padangusthasana D.

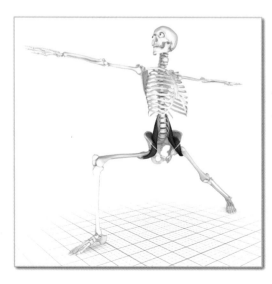

Closed Chain
(Insertion fixed, origin moving):

Flexes the trunk, anteverts (tilts forward) the pelvis, straightens and supports the lumbar spine, e.g., Virabhadrasana II.

Awakening

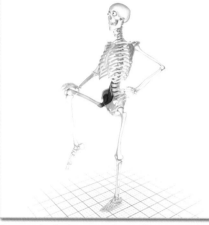

Open-chain isometric resistance to the femur flexing.

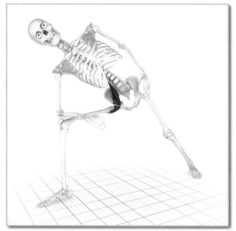

Closed-chain isometric resistance to the trunk flexing.

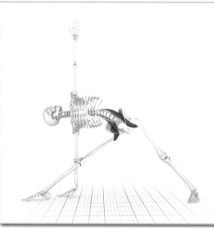

Concentric contraction in standing poses.

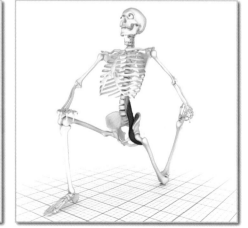

Eccentric contraction in lunging poses.

Contracted

Utthita Trikonasana optimally contracts the psoas major portion of the iliopsoas muscle. Contraction in this posture anteverts the pelvis. This action draws the hamstrings' origin (the ischial tuberosity) away from their insertion (lower leg), and accentuates their stretch.

Twisted variations of Utthita Trikonasana preferentially contract the iliacus portion of the iliopsoas and complete its awakening.

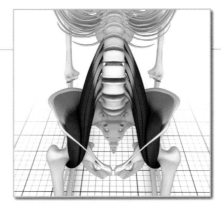

Stretched

Ustrasana stretches the iliopsoas by contracting the hip and trunk extensors, including the gluteus maximus. The stretch is accentuated by contracting the quadriceps (including the rectus femoris, which is eccentrically contracted).

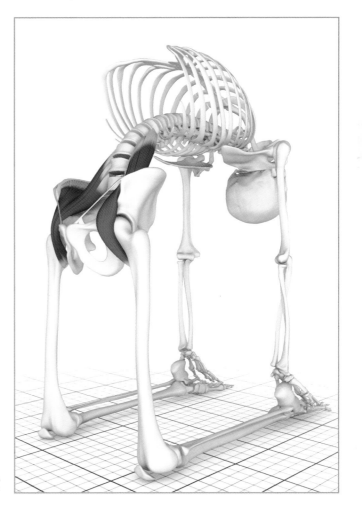

Chapter 2

Gluteus Maximus

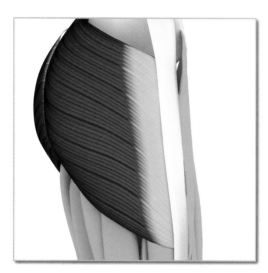

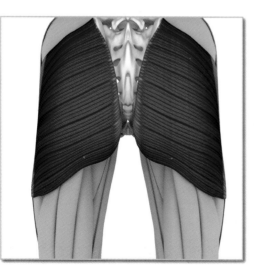

The gluteus maximus stands out as the largest and most posterior of four muscles located on the outside of the pelvis. It is a single muscle divided into two insertions: one on the outside of the proximal femur bone and one on a strap-like structure on the outside of the thigh called the iliotibial band. Contracting the gluteus maximus extends and outwardly rotates the femur. Fibers attached to the iliotibial band tense it and assist in moving the knee. The gluteus maximus functions as a mono- and polyarticular muscle. Tightness of the gluteus maximus limits forward bending at the hips, such as in Uttanasana.

Like the iliopsoas, the gluteus maximus works unconsciously during standing and walking. Many important Yoga postures awaken the gluteus maximus, including standing poses, back bends, and forward bends. Tightness limits forward bends, and weakness limits back bends.

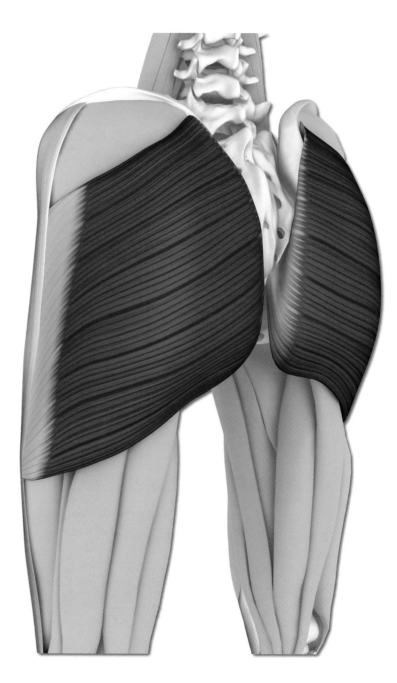

Gluteus Maximus (GLOO-te-us MAK-si-mus)

Origin

Outer posterior surface of the illium, posterior surface of the sacrum and coccyx, and the aponeurosis of the erector spinae muscles of the back.

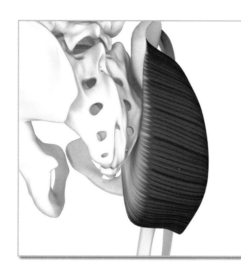

Insertion

1) Gluteal tuberosity on the lateral surface of the proximal femur below the greater trochanter.

2) Iliotibial band (inserts onto Gerdys' tubercle on the front of the proximal tibia).

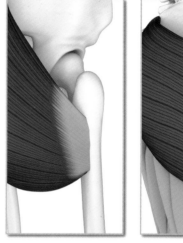
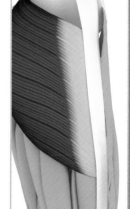

Innervation & Chakra Illuminated

Inferior gluteal nerve (lumbar spinal nerve 5 and sacral spinal nerves 1 and 2).

Chakra illuminated: First.

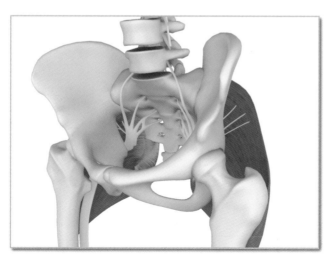

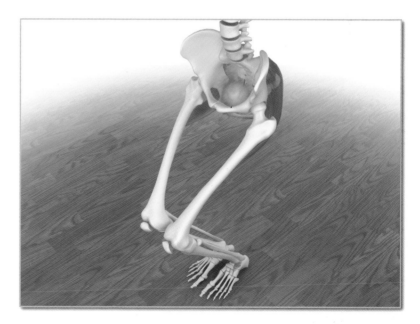

Gluteus Maximus (GLOO-te-us MAK-si-mus)

Synergists

Semimembranosus, semitendinosis, biceps femoris, quadratus lumborum, and adductor magnus.

Antagonists

Iliopsoas, rectus femoris, and pectineus.

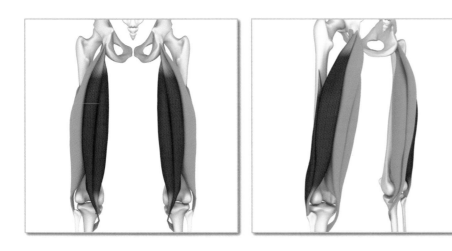
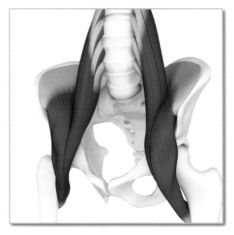
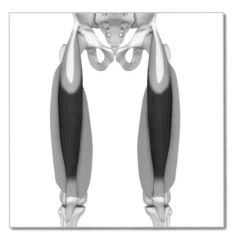

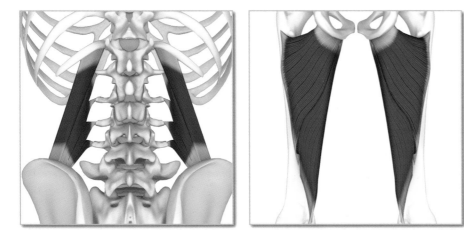
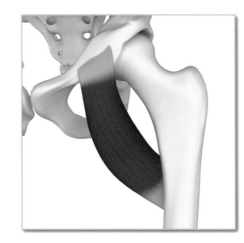

Action

Extends and externally rotates the hip. Upper fibers assist to abduct the thigh. Assists to stabilize fully the extended knee (via the iliotibial band).

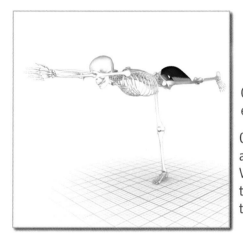

Open-chain contraction extends and externally rotates the hip joint.

Contracting the gluteus maximus lifts and externally rotates the back leg in Virabhadrasana III. The fibers inserting on the iliotibial band also assist in stabilizing the straight knee.

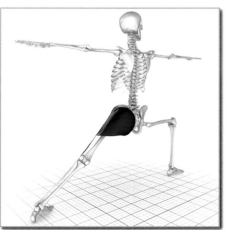

Closed-chain contraction extends the trunk in Virabhadrasana II.

Awakening

The gluteus maximus can be eccentrically contracted in Padangusthasana, stretching and strengthening it.

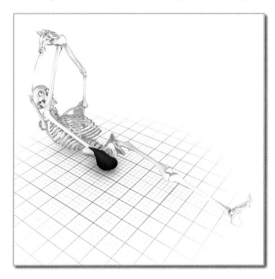

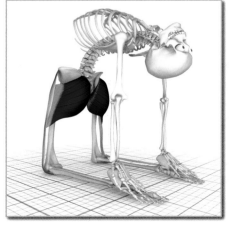

Closed-chain contraction of the gluteus maximus in Ustrasana extends the trunk.

Gluteus Maximus (GLOO-te-us MAK-si-mus)

Contracted

Purvottanasana: The gluteus maximus contracts in this Asana. Its external rotation component is counteracted by contraction of the gluteus medius (anterior fibers), tensor fascia lata, and adductor group. (Accentuate this by pressing down the ball of the foot.)

Stretched

Uttanasana: The gluteus maximus stretches in this and other Asanas that flex the trunk and hips.

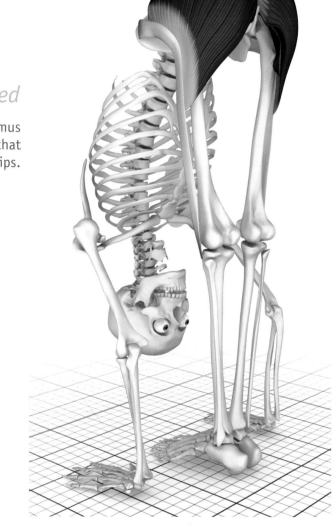

Chapter3

Gluteus Medius

The gluteus medius presents a medium-sized, fan-shaped muscle located forward of the gluteus maximus, which partially covers it. The gluteus medius inserts on the tip of the greater trochanter (a protuberance on the proximal femur to which muscles attach). The gluteus medius covers the gluteus minimus.

Direction and placement of muscle fibers determines the movement produced by contraction. Anterior fibers internally rotate and middle fibers abduct the femur. When the femur is fixed in place, as in one-legged standing poses, contracting the gluteus medius tilts the pelvis, maintaining balance.

We are largely unaware of the gluteus medius, though it is constantly active and balances the pelvis when standing and walking. Contract it in back bends to counterbalance the external rotation of the hips produced by contraction of the gluteus maximus.

Tightness in the gluteus medius limits postures that require extensive external rotation of the femur at the hip (e.g., Lotus posture). Weakness limits one-legged standing poses.

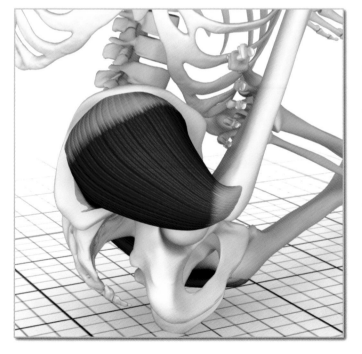

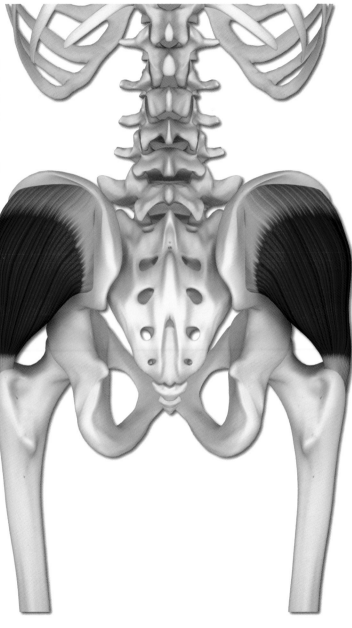

Gluteus Medius (GLOO -te-us ME-de-us)

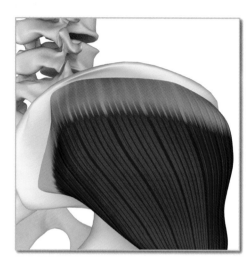

Origin

Outer surface of the ilium below the iliac crest and anterior to the gluteus maximus' origin.

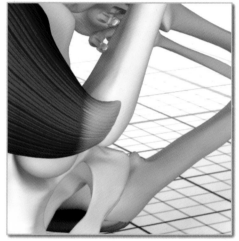

Insertion

Superior surface of greater trochanter of the proximal femur.

Gluteus Minimus

This see-through image of the gluteus medius illustrates the position of the gluteus minimus, which has a similar function.

Origin

Outer surface of the ilium below and anterior to the gluteus medius' origin.

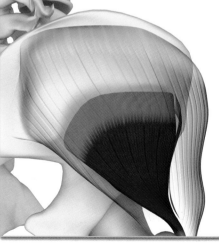

Insertion

Anterior portion of the greater trochanter.

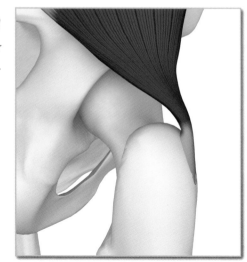

Synergists

Gluteus minimus, tensor fascia lata, and piriformis.

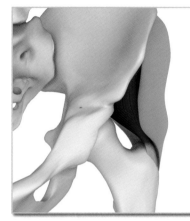
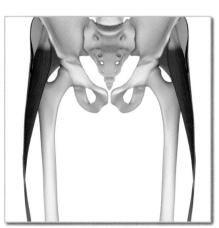
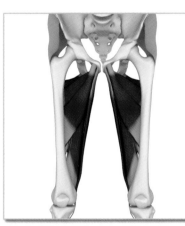
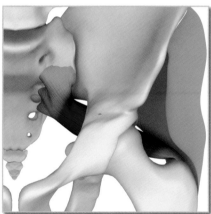

Antagonists

Adductor group and quadratus femoris.

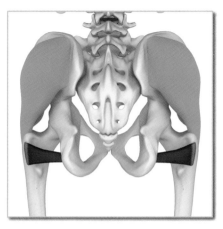

Innervation & Chakra Illuminated

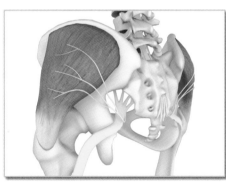

Superior gluteal nerve (lumbar spinal nerves 4 and 5 and sacral spinal nerve 1).

Chakra illuminated: First.

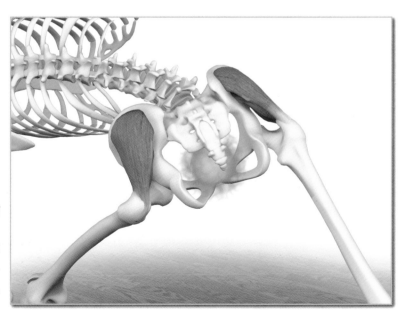

Gluteus Medius (GLOO -te-us ME-de-us)

Action

Abducts and internally rotates the hip. Stabilizes the pelvis during walking. Posterior fibers may externally rotate the thigh.

The gluteus medius contracts and abducts the bent leg in Janu Sirsasana. Anterior fibers also medially rotate the thigh, protecting the knee.

The gluteus medius contracts and abducts the straight leg, lifting it in Ardha Chandrasana.

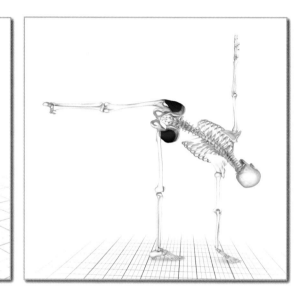

Awakening

Contracting the gluteus medius in Marichyasana IV accentuates the twist. This isometric contraction awakens the gluteus medius.

Contracting the gluteus medius in the back leg of Parivrtta Trikonasana accentuates the twist from the trunk by rotating the femur.

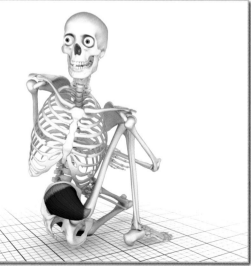
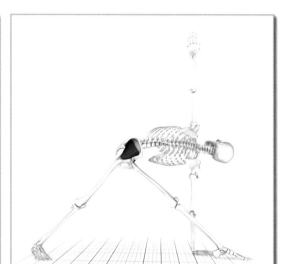

Contracted

Urdhva Danurasana: Contracting the anterior fibers of the gluteus medius internally rotates the hips and releases stress at the sacroiliac joint created by contracting the gluteus maximus (to extend the hip).

Stretched

Vatayanasana: Externally rotating the hip stretches the gluteus medius (especially the anterior fibers). All poses with a Lotus component to the hips (external rotation) accomplish this.

Chapter4
Tensor Fascia Lata

This small polyarticular muscle originates at the iliac crest in front of the gluteus medius, assisting it with internal rotation of the hip. Inserting on the iliotibial band, it also works with the anterior fibers of the gluteus maximus to extend the knee.

Tightness in the tensor fascia lata limits postures that externally rotate the hip, such as Padmasana.

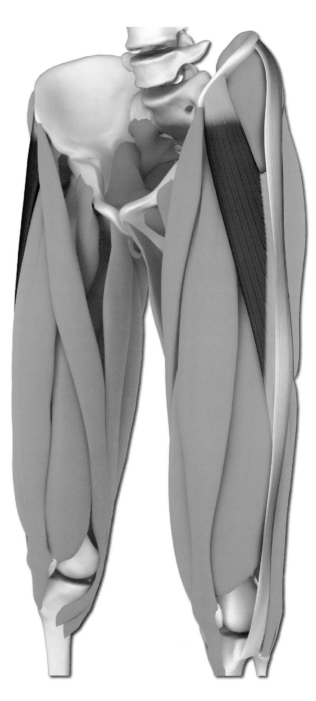

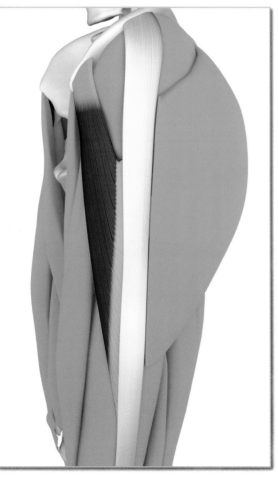

Tensor Fascia Lata (TEN-sor FASH-e-a LA-te)

Origin

Anterior portion of the outside of the iliac crest and the anterior superior iliac spine.

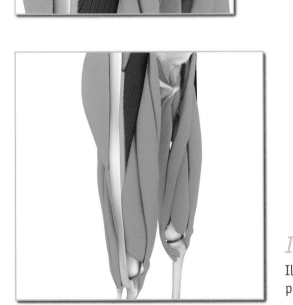

Innervation & Chakra Illuminated

Superior gluteal nerve (lumbar nerves 4 and 5 and sacral nerve 1).

Chakra illuminated: First.

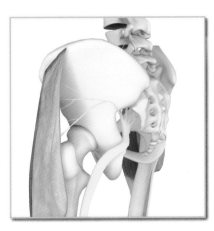

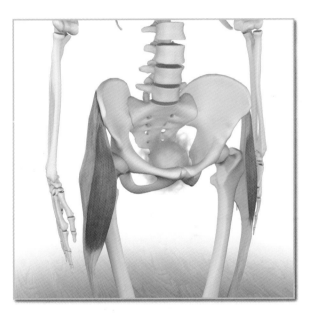

Insertion

Iliotibial band (and from there to the anterolateral proximal tibia).

Tensor Fascia Lata (TEN-sor FASH-e-a LA-te)

Antagonists

Hamstrings, adductor group, and gluteus maximus (femoral insertion).

Synergists

Quadriceps, iliopsoas, and anterior portion of gluteus maximus (iliotibial band insertion), gluteus medius.

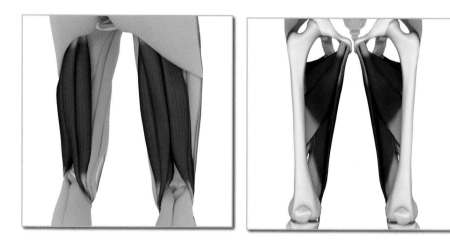

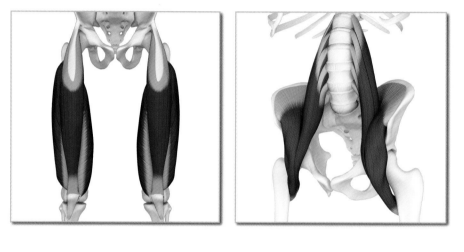

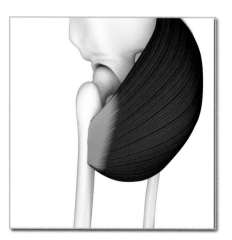

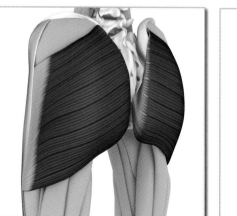

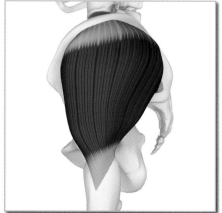

Action

Flexes, internally rotates, and abducts the hip; supports the femur on the tibia during standing.

Open-chain contraction in Parsvottonasana and Urdhva Danurasana turns the thighs inward and straightens the knees.

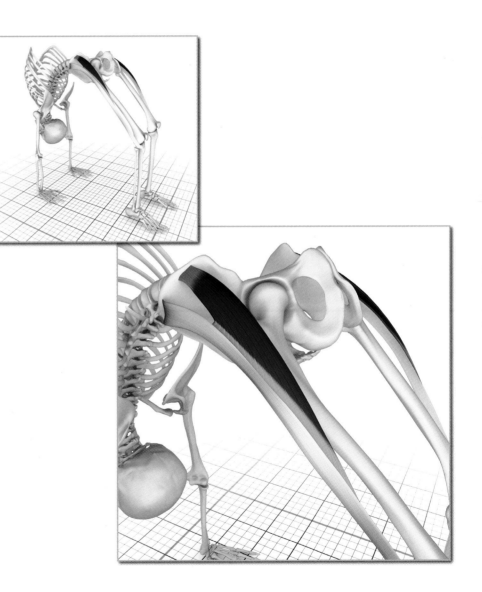

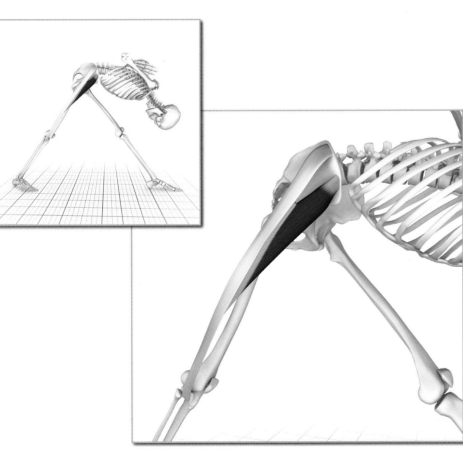

Tensor Fascia Lata (TEN-sor FASH-e-a LA-te)

Stretched

Padmasana stretches the tensor fascia lata. Eccentric contraction in this pose facilitates this, awakening the muscle.

Contracted

Contracting the tensor fascia lata stabilizes the lifted leg in Ardha Chandrasana.

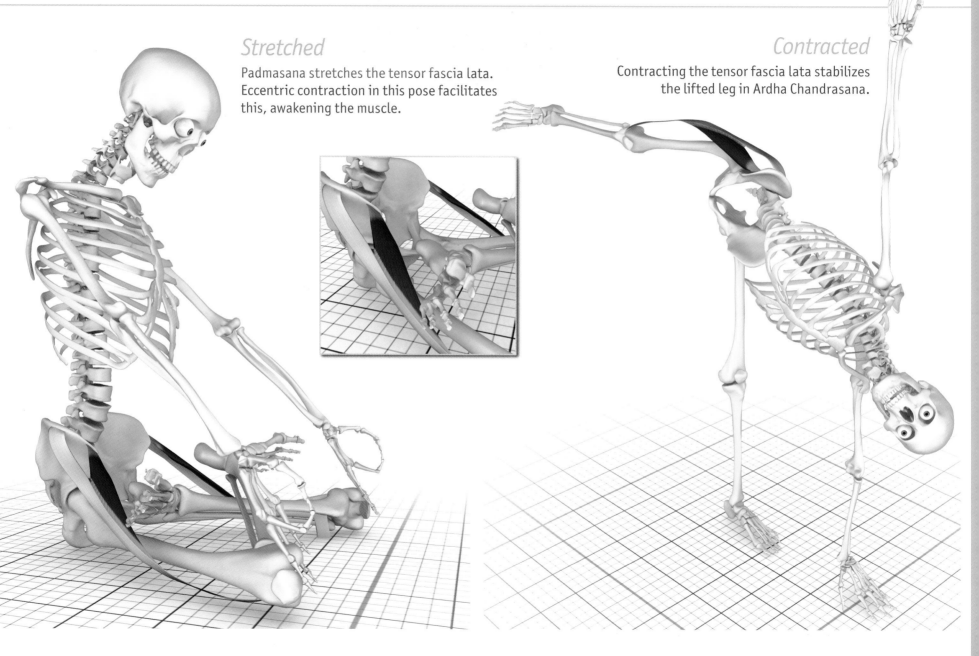

Chapter 5a

Pectineus

The pectineus is the proximal muscle in the adductor group. It is a flat rectangular muscle originating from the front of the pelvic girdle and inserting on the inside of the proximal femur. It is monoarticular.

Tightness in the pectineus limits the depth of poses like Baddha Konasana.

Weakness limits Gomukhasana B. Contraction accentuates Mula Bandha.

Awareness of the pectineus awakens its neighboring adductor muscles, the brevis and longus.

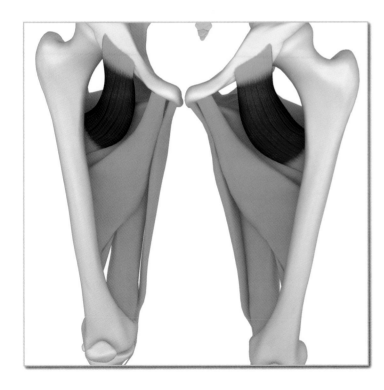

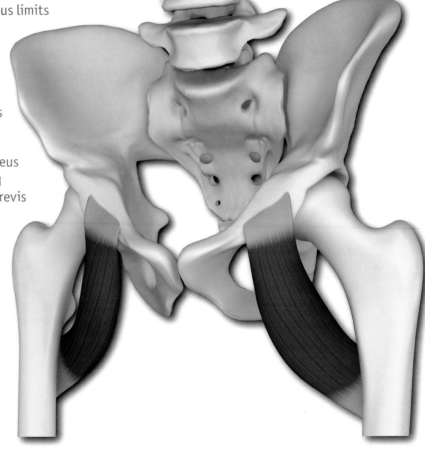

Pectineus (pec-ti-NEUS)

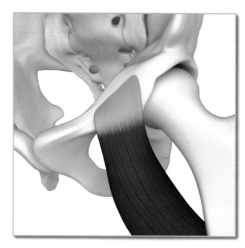

Origin

Pecten (a bulge) of the pubic bone on the iliopubic ramus, lateral to the pubic symphysis (front view).

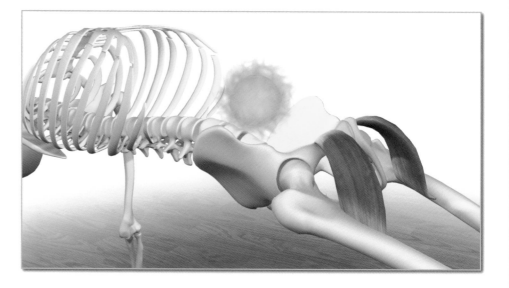

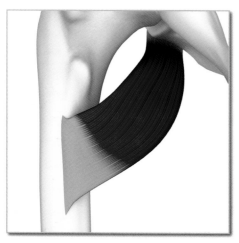

Insertion

Pectineal line extending from the lesser trochanter to the linea aspera on the inside of the proximal femur (back view).

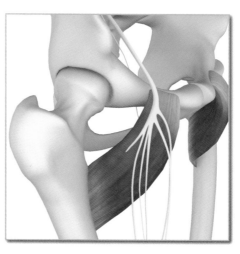

Innervation & Chakra Illuminated

Femoral nerve (lumbar spinal nerves 3 and 4) obturator nerve (lumbar spinal nerves 2, 3, and 4).

Chakra illuminated: Second.

Antagonists

Gluteus medius, gluteus minimus, tensor fascia lata, and piriformis.

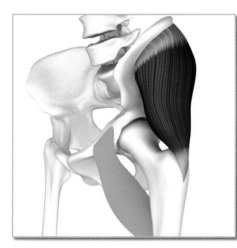 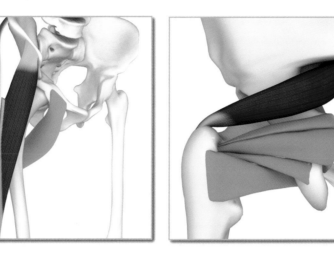

Synergists

Adductor group, illiopsoas, and quadratus femoris.

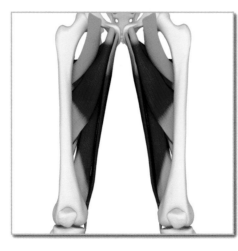 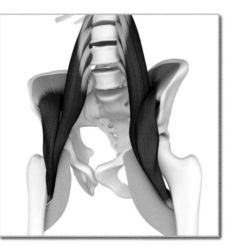 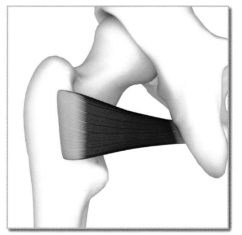

Pectineus (pec-ti-NEUS)

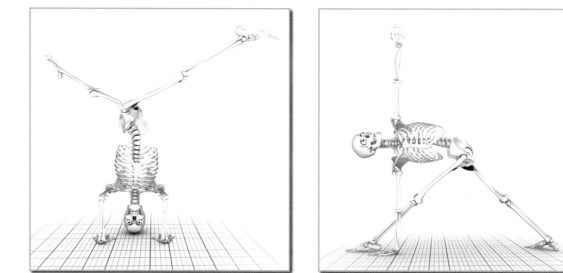

Action

Adducts, flexes, and internally rotates the hip.

The pectineus contracts in Parivrttaikapada Sirsasana, adducting both femurs and assisting the iliopsoas, flexing the forward hip. This same principle applies in Parivrtta Trikonasana.

Awakening

Baddha Konasana awakens the pectineus. Isometric, eccentric contraction accentuates this.

Closed-chain contraction of the front leg pectineus draws the pelvis (and trunk) forward in Parsvottanasana.

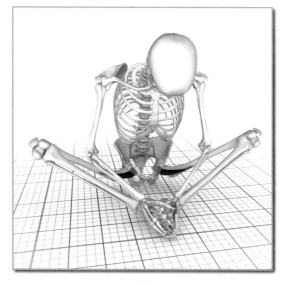

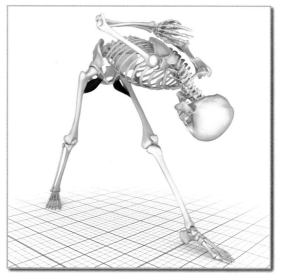

Stretched

Baddha Konasana: The pectineus is at full stretch in the upright version of this Asana.

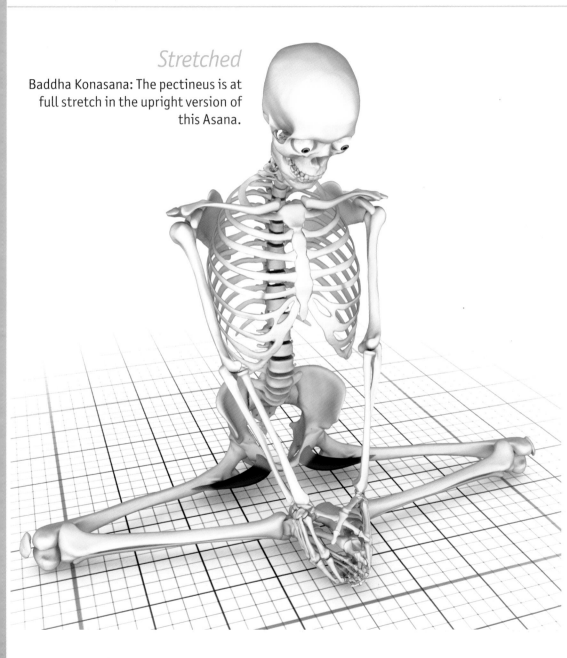

Contracted

Bakasana: Contracting the adductor group stabilizes this Asana.

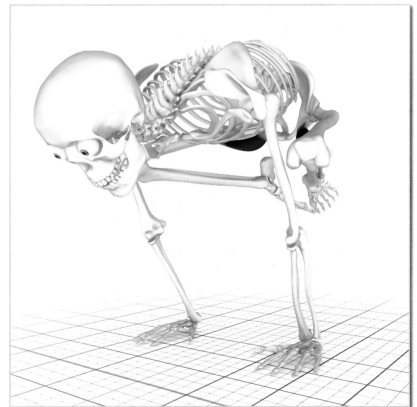

Chapter 5b

Adductor Magnus

This is the largest and most posterior of the adductor group. It originates from the back of the pelvis and inserts along the length of the inside of the femur. A hole or "hiatus" in the distal region of its insertion allows passage of the femoral blood vessels.

Its posterior location means that it functions to adduct and extend the thigh backward. It is a synergist to the gluteus maximus, assisting it in back-bending postures such as Urdhva Danurasana. Tightness limits poses such as front splits. Weakness limits Bakasana. Contraction of the adductor magnus accentuates Mula Bandha.

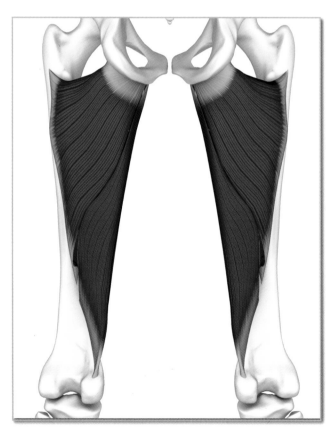

Posterior

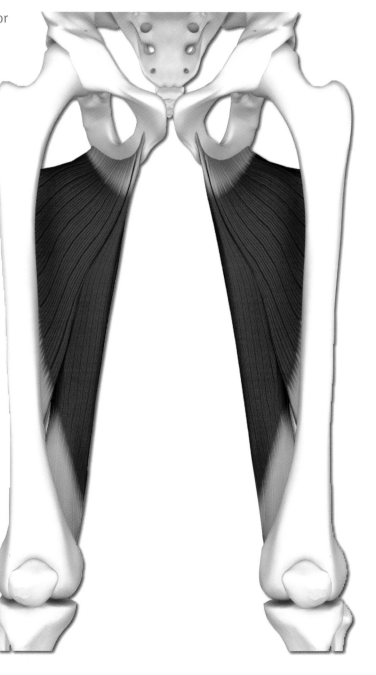

Adductor Magnus (ad-DUK-tor MAG-nus)

Origin

Anterior section:
Ischiopubic ramus.

Posterior section:
Ischial tuberosity.

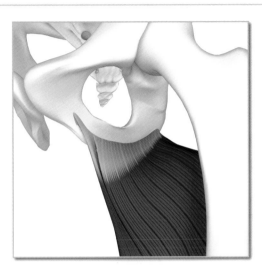

Insertion

1) Anterior section: Linea aspera on the back of the middle third of the femur.

2) Posterior section: Medial epicondyle on the inside of the distal femur above the knee joint.

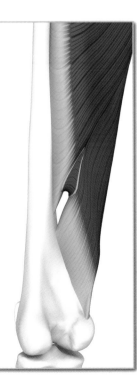

Innervation & Chakra Illuminated

Anterior fibers: Obturator nerve (lumbar spinal nerves 2, 3, and 4).
Posterior fibers: Tibial portion of sciatic nerve (lumbar spinal nerves 3, 4, and 5).

Chakra illuminated:
Upper part of first, lower part of second.

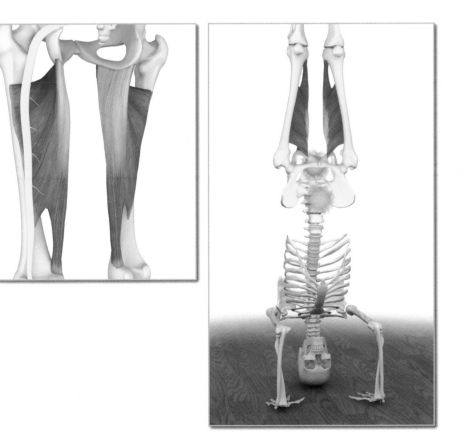

Adductor Magnus (ad-DUK-tor MAG-nus)

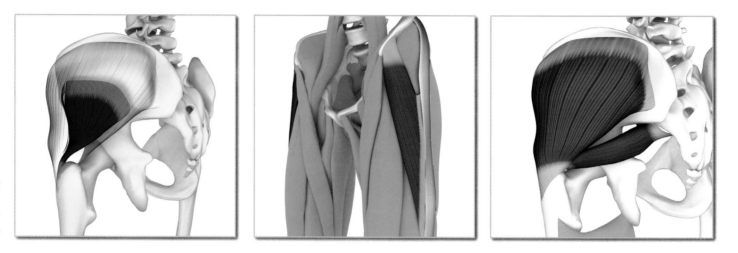

Antagonists

Gluteus medius, gluteus minimus, tensor fascia lata, and piriformis.

Synergists

Adductor group and quadratus femoris.

Action

Adducts the hip. Posterior fibers extend and externally rotate the hip.

Contracting the adductor magnus squeezes the thighs together in Parsva Bakasana.

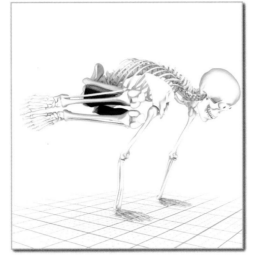

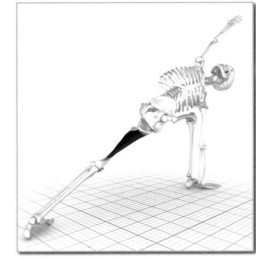

Contracting the adductor magnus assists the gluteus maximus, extending and externally rotating the back leg in Parivrtta Parsvakonasana.

Awakening

Upavistha Konasana stretches and awakens the adductor magnus by abducting and flexing the hip.

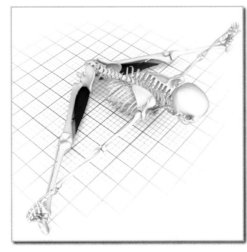

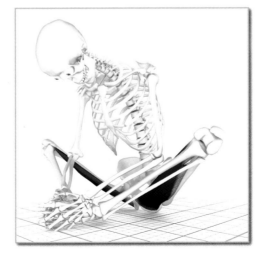

Baddha Konasa stretches and awakens the adductor magnus through isometric eccentric contraction.

Adductor Magnus (ad-DUK-tor MAG-nus)

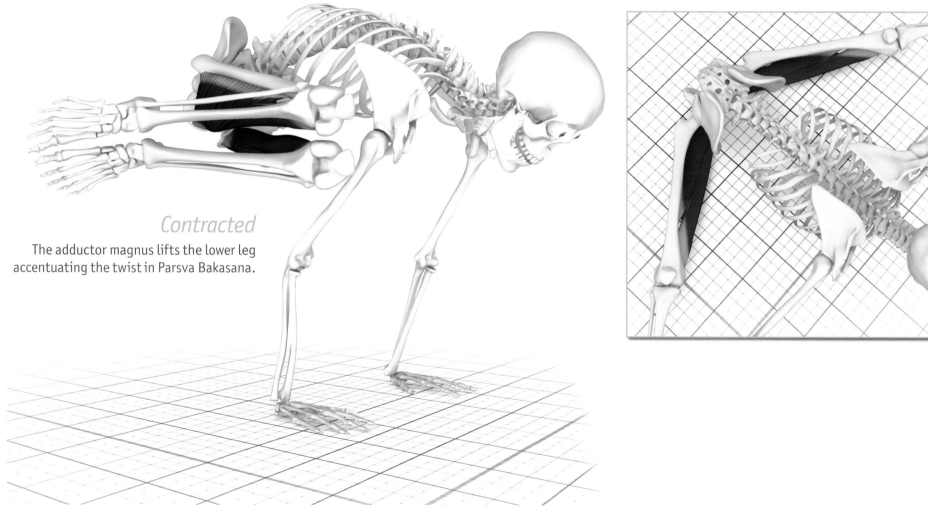

Stretched

The adductor magnus and the entire adductor group stretches in Upavistha Konasana (the more distal and posterior muscles are preferentially stretched).

Contracted

The adductor magnus lifts the lower leg accentuating the twist in Parsva Bakasana.

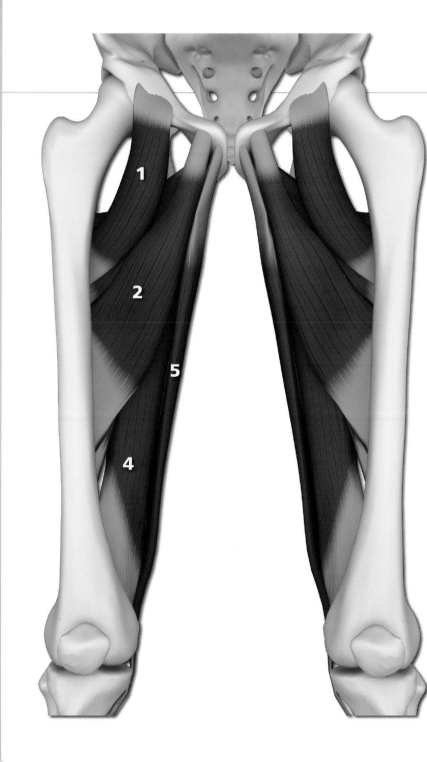

1
pectineus

2
longus

3
brevis

4
magnus

5
gracilis

Adductor Group

Tightness of the adductor group causes the knees to be higher in seated postures, such as Baddha Konasana and Siddhasana. Higher knees means a higher center of gravity. Holding a seated posture where the center of gravity is higher requires more muscular effort. Lowering the knees makes these postures easier to maintain. Releasing tightness in the adductor group assists in this process.

Facilitated stretching of the adductor group is illustrated here. Begin by placing the legs into Baddha Konasana and then attempt to adduct them while resisting them with the elbows. Contract the adductors isometrically for a few moments and then draw them out to length by lowering the knees.

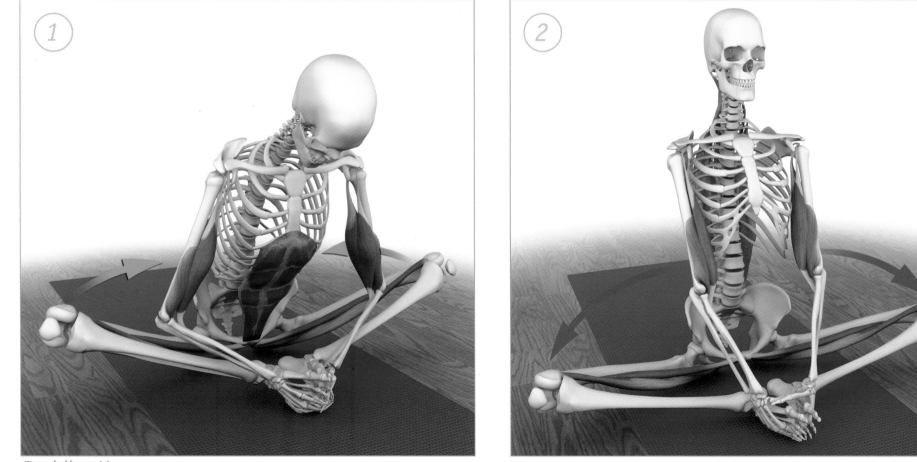

Baddha Konasana

Chapter 6
External Rotators

Piriformis & Quadratus Femoris

Piriformis (piri-FOR-mus):

This is a pyramid-shaped muscle originating from the inside of the pelvis at the sacrum. The piriformis wraps around the ilium and inserts on the tip of the greater trochanter on the proximal femur.

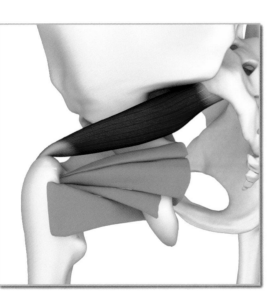

This creates a pulley effect multiplying the piriformis' force — much like what occurs with the iliopsoas as it curves over the front of the pelvis. The sciatic nerve runs behind the piriformis and can be irritated by tightness or inflammation of this muscle, a phenomenon known as "piriformis syndrome." The piriformis acts in open- and closed-chain fashions. When its origin (the sacrum) is fixed, contraction produces external rotation and abduction of the femur. When the femur is fixed, contraction tilts the pelvis backward. Tightness in the piriformis limits internal rotation of the thigh in certain seated twists and in twisted standing poses.

Quadratus Femoris (KWA-drat-us fe-MOR-us):

This is the most distal of the external rotators. It is a quadrangular-shaped muscle originating from above the ischial tuberosity and inserting on the greater trochanter of the proximal femur. It is a synergist to the piriformis in external rotation of the femur. It is also an adductor of the femur and opposes the piriformis' capacity to abduct. Combined contraction of the two muscles externally rotates the thigh.

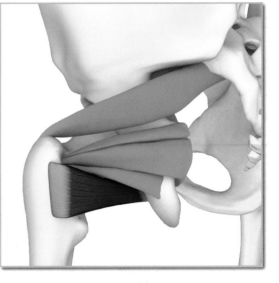

Tightness in the quadratus femoris limits internal rotation of the femur in certain seated twists and in twisted standing poses. Contraction accentuates the effect of other seated twists and non-twisted standing poses. Awakening the piriformis and quadratus femoris muscles brings awareness to the neighboring gamelli and obturators (the other external rotators of the hip).

Piriformis & Quadratus Femoris

Origin-Piriformis

Inside surface of sacrum and sacrotuberous ligament.

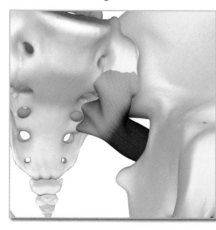

Origin-Quadratus Femoris

Lateral surface of ischial tuberosity.

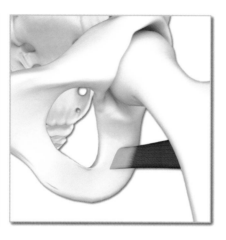

Innervation & Chakra Illuminated

Piriformis: Nerve to piriformis (sacral nerves 1 and 2).

Quadratus Femoris: Nerve to quadratus femoris (lumbar nerves 4 and 5 and sacral nerve 1).

Chakra illuminated: First.

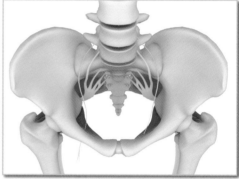

Insertion

Piriformis: Tip of greater trochanter.

Quadratus femoris: Posterior surface of the femur at the level of the greater trochanter.

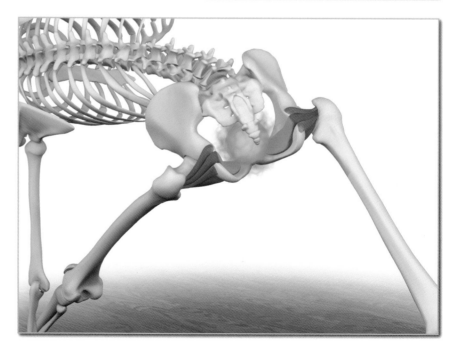

Antagonists-Piriformis

Adductor group and gluteus medius (anterior fibers).

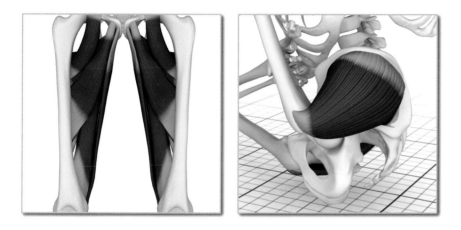

Synergists-Piriformis

Gluteus medius (lateral and posterior fibers), gluteus minimus, and tensor fascia lata.

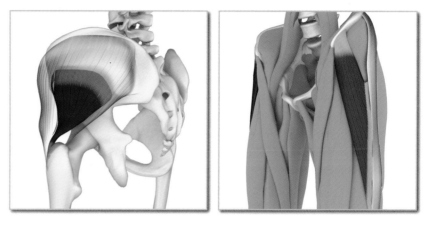

Antagonists-Quadratus Femoris

Gluteus medius (anterior fibers), gluteus minimus, and tensor fascia lata.

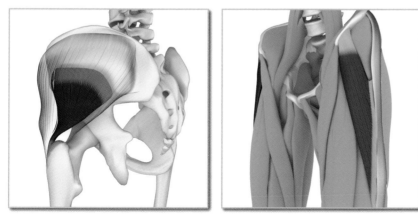

Synergists-Quadratus Femoris

Adductor group.

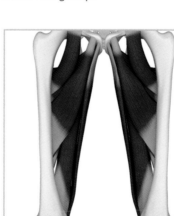
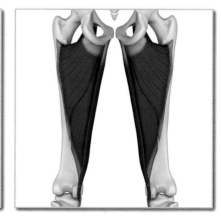

Piriformis & Quadratus Femoris

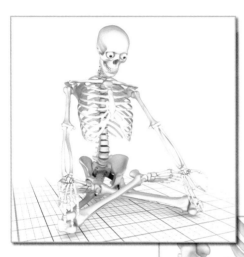

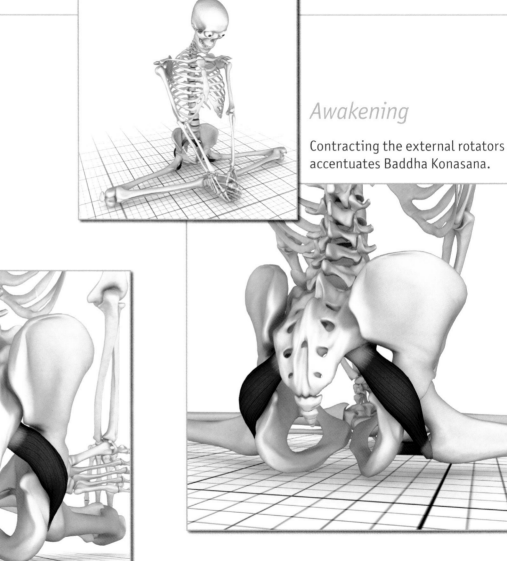

Awakening

Contracting the external rotators accentuates Baddha Konasana.

Action

The piriformis externally rotates and abducts the hip. The quadratus femoris externally rotates and adducts the hip.

Closed chain of the piriformis contraction tilts the pelvis backward.

The external rotators position the hips in external rotation for Padmasana.

Contracted

Utthita Hasta Padangusthasana B: All external rotators of the hip contract in this Asana. The piriformis also assists the lateral fibers of the gluteus medius, abducting the femur.

Stretched

Marichyasana III: Contracting the internal rotators of the hip (tensor fascia lata and anterior fibers of gluteus medius) in this Asana stretches the external rotators.

Chapter7
Quadriceps

The quadriceps muscle forms the front of the thigh. Its name, derived from Latin, means "four headed." It is a four-part muscle combining to form the quadriceps tendon, which inserts on the patella (kneecap). The patellar tendon is a functional continuation of the quadriceps tendon, inserting on the front of the proximal tibia. The patella is a "sesamoid" bone (stone-like). This refers to a bone within a tendon. Acting as a fulcrum, it increases the force produced by contraction of the quadriceps when straightening the knee.

The rectus femoris – unique in that it originates from the front of the pelvis at the anterior-inferior iliac spine – continues on the front of the thigh, covering the vastus intermedius and combining with the other quadriceps to insert on the patella. It works as a polyarticular muscle. Force produced by its contraction results in a combination of two possible movements: flexion of the hip and extension of the knee. The other three heads of the quadriceps are monoarticular and only act to straighten the knee.

The quadriceps are key muscles in Yoga. Contracting them directly stretches the hamstrings when seated or in standing poses. They also straighten the knees in backbends, lifting the body.

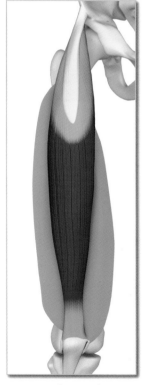

rectus femoris

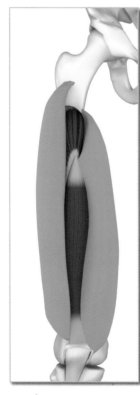

vastus intermedius

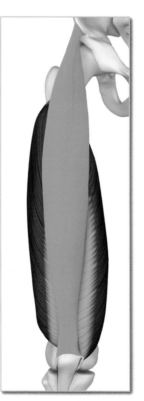

vastus medialis
vastus lateralis

Quadriceps (KWA-dra-seps)

Origin

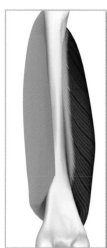

Vastus Medialis

Proximal two-thirds of the anterior femur.

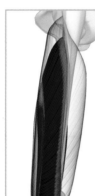

Vastus Intermedius

Lateral portion of proximal femur in region of greater trochanter (seen through the vastus lateralis).

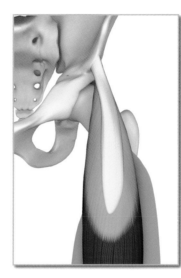

Origin–Rectus Femoris

Anterior inferior iliac spine.

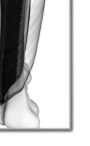

Vastus Lateralis

Lateral portion of proximal femur in region of greater trochanter.

Insertion–All

Quadriceps tendon: Superior surface of patella (and on to the anterior proximal tibia via the patellar tendon).

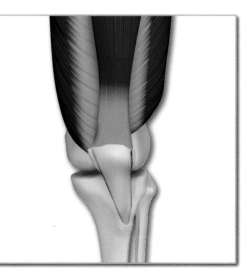

Quadriceps

Innervation & Chakra Illuminated

Femoral nerve (lumbar nerves 2, 3, and 4).

Chakra illuminated:

Second.

Synergists

Iliopsoas, tensor fascia lata.

Antagonists

Hamstrings, gastrocnemius, sartorius, gracilis.

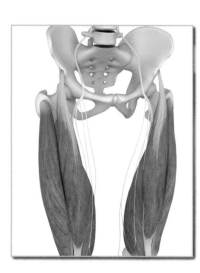

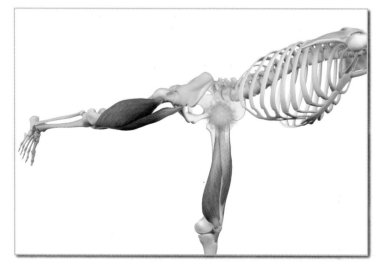

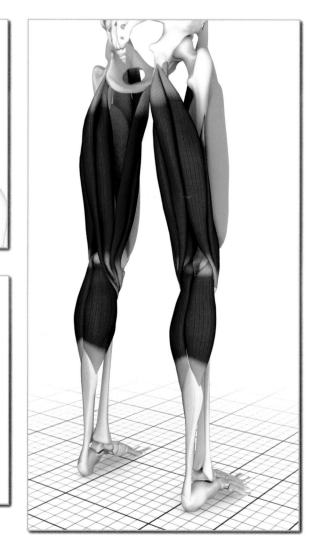

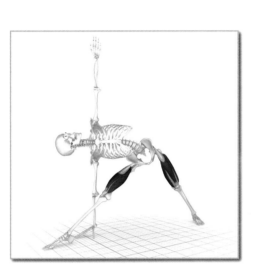

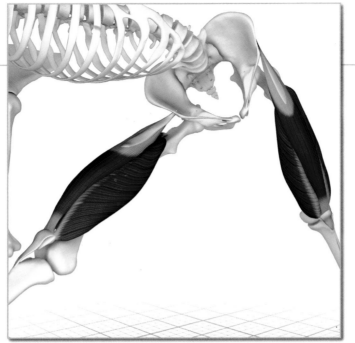

Action

Extends the knee.

Rectus femoris also flexes the hip.
The quadriceps contract, extending the knee
and flexing the hip (rectus femoris) in Utthita
Trikonasana.

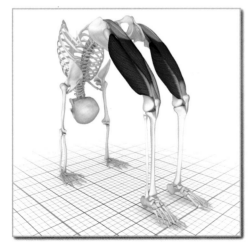

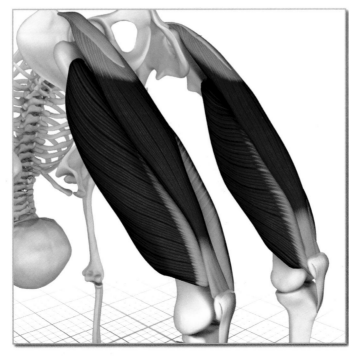

Awakening

The vastus lateralis, medialis, and intermedius
contract, straightening the knee in Urdhva
Danurasana. The rectus femoris stretches and
contracts (eccentric contraction).

Quadriceps

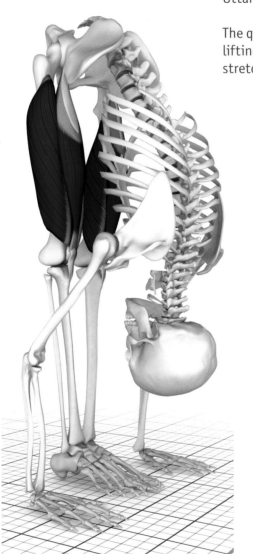

Contracted

Uttanasana:

The quadriceps contract in this forward bend, lifting the patella, straightening the knee, and stretching their antagonists (the hamstrings).

Stretched

Trianga Mukhaikapada Paschimottanasana:

Bending the knee stretches the vastus lateralis, medialis, and intermedius. The rectus femoris relaxes due to the flexed position of the hip. The straight leg quadriceps contract, stretching the corresponding hamstings.

Knee Biomechanics

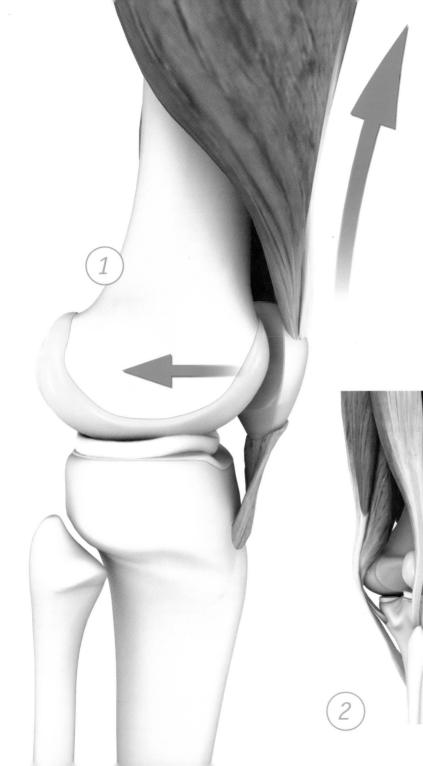

Contracting the quadriceps draws the patella upward and against the anterior femur into a groove between the femoral condyles. The patella fits congruently into the intercondylar groove, stabilizing the standing leg. In this way, the patella acts as a fulcrum for knee extension.

The flexors of the knee counterbalance the extension force of the quadriceps. These images illustrate how the knee flexors and extensors oppose each other, stabilizing the knee.

It is important to avoid hyperextension or "locking" of the knee during standing poses. This can overstretch the hamstrings and creates unhealthy stress on the knee's articular cartilage.

Contracting the knee flexors helps to avoid hyperextending the knee. For example, pressing down the ball of the foot contracts the gastroctnemius, stabilizing the knee.

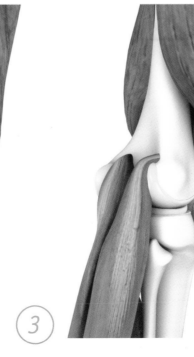

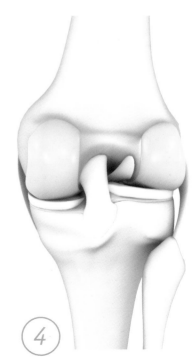

Sartorius (sar-TOR-e-us)

The sartorius is a long strap-like muscle originating from the anterior superior iliac spine and inserting on the upper medial surface of the tibia. This muscle flexes, abducts, and externally rotates the thigh, as in Siddhasana, Padmasana, Vrksasana, and Janu Sirsasana. In fact, the Latin translation for sartorius is "tailor," because tailors used to sit cross-legged. The femoral nerve innervates the sartorius, stimulating the second Chakra.

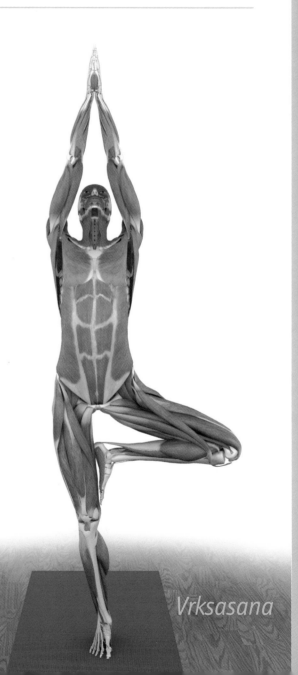

Vrksasana

Chapter 8
Hamstrings

Biceps Femoris (BI-seps fe-MOR-us)

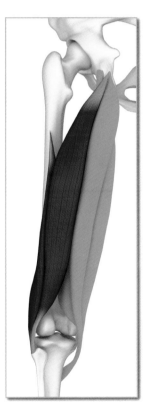

The biceps femoris is a two-headed fusiform-shaped muscle. One head originates from the ischial tuberosity, the other from the back of the femur. Both heads combine to form a single tendon insertion on the head of the fibula bone at the lateral side of the knee. It can be palpated as a cord in this region.

The biceps femoris flexes the straight knee and outwardly rotates the lower leg (in the bent knee). Its rotary action accentuates twisting postures, such as Marichyasana III. Tightness in this muscle limits forward bends and certain standing poses, especially those involving internal rotation of the leg.

Semitendinosus (sem-e-ten-di-NO-sus)
Semimembranosus (sem-e-mem-bruh-NO-sus)

These two muscles make up the inner hamstrings. The semimembranosus has a flattened wide belly. The semitendinosus is fusiform in shape (tapered at both ends), with the distal end forming a long tendon. Both muscles originate from the ischial tuberosity. They have separate insertions on the proximal tibia, one on the inside of the back of the tibia (semimembranosus) and one on the inside of the front of the tibia (semitendinosus). The semitendinosus insertion combines with the sartorius and gracilis muscles to form a broad duckfoot-like insertion on the anterior tibia called the pes anserinus.

The semimembranosus and semitendinosus flex the straight knee, inwardly rotating the lower leg in the bent knee. This rotary component accentuates seated twists, but in the opposite direction of the biceps femoris. Contraction of these muscles also assists the gluteus maximus in extension of the thigh at the hip, as in Virabhadrasana III. Tightness in this muscle limits forward bends and certain standing poses, especially those involving external rotation of the leg.

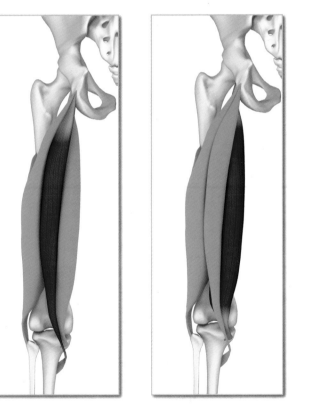

Semitendinosus   Semimembranosus

Hamstrings

Origin-Biceps Femoris

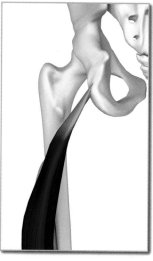

Long head:

Ischial tuberosity (long head origin is shared with the semitendinosus.)

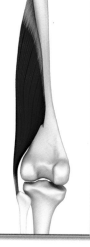

Short head:

Linea aspera on the upper two-thirds of the posterior femur.

Insertion-Biceps Femoris

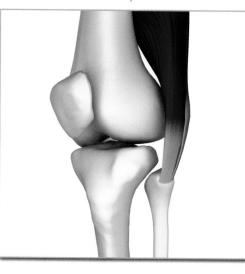

Head of fibula.

Origin-Semimembranosus & Semitendinosus

Ischial tuberosity: (semitendinosus origin is shared with the long head of the biceps femoris).

Insertion-Semimembranosus & Semitendinosus

1) Semimembranosus: Posteromedial surface of proximal tibia. Some fibers join to form the oblique popliteal ligament and attach to the posterior medial meniscus.

2) Semitendinosus: Upper inner surface of the proximal tibia (contributes to pes anserinus).

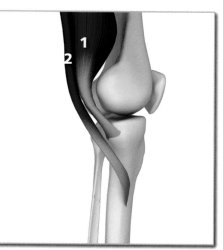

Innervation & Chakra Illuminated

Biceps femoris

1) Long head: Tibial portion of the sciatic nerve (sacral nerves 1 and 2).
2) Short head: Fibular portion of sciatic nerve (lumbar nerve 5 and sacral nerves 1 and 2).

Semimembranosus semitendinosus tibial nerve (lumbar nerve 5 and sacral nerve 1).

Chakra illuminated: First.

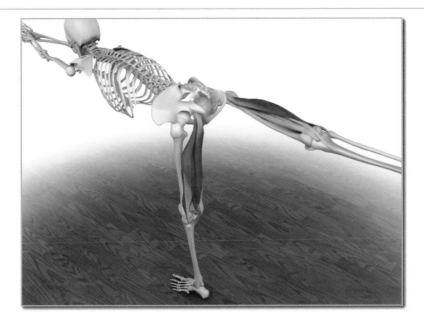

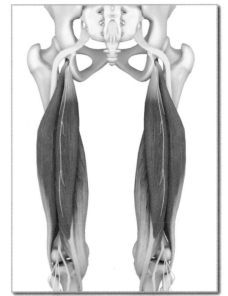

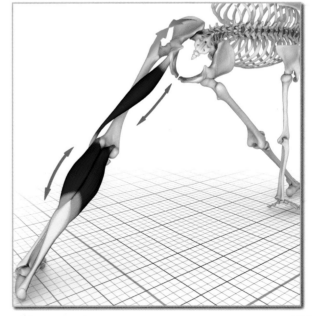

Gluteus maximus (illustrated by green arrows) extending the hip and knee, stretching the long head of the biceps femoris (and gastrocnemius).

Hamstrings

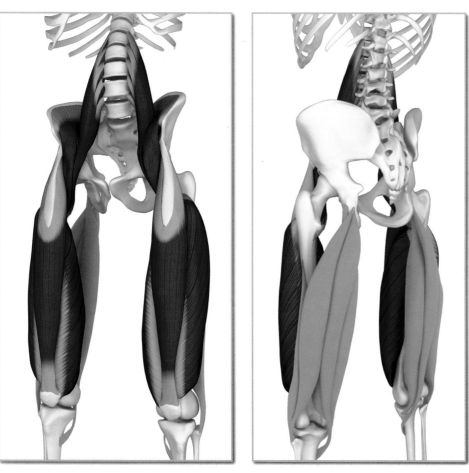

Antagonists

Quadriceps and iliopsoas.

Synergists

Gluteus maximus, sartorius, gracilis, and gastrocnemius.

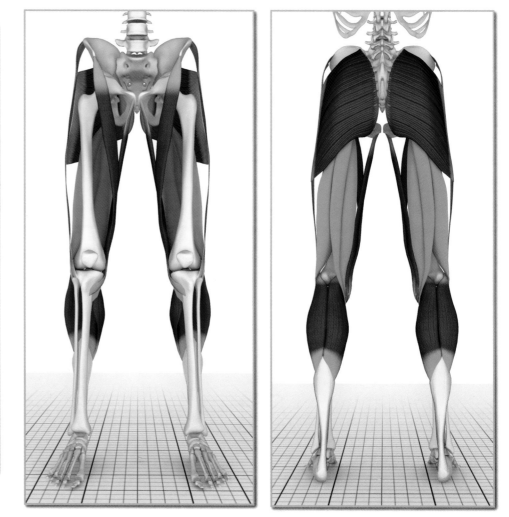

Front View (Anterior)

Back View (Posterior)

Biceps Femoris

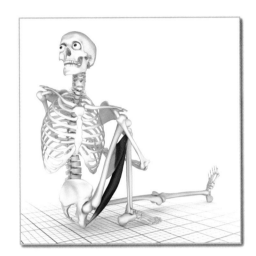

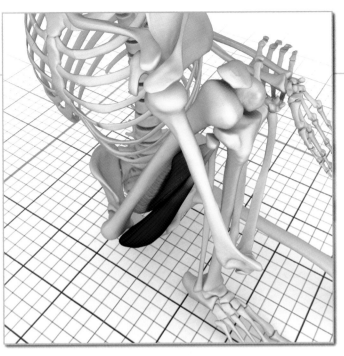

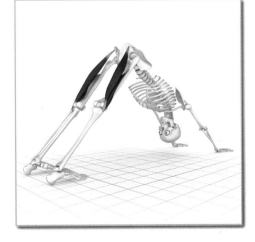

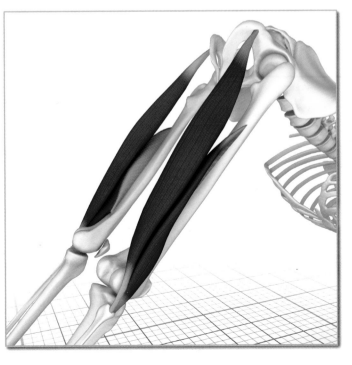

Action

Flexes the knee and extends the hip (long head). Externally rotates the tibia in the flexed knee.

The biceps femoris contracts, flexing the knee and externally rotating the tibia in Marichyasana III. This external rotation manifests as internal rotation of the hip, accentuating the twist of the trunk.

Awakening

Adho Mukha Svanasana stretches and awakens the biceps femoris.

Semimembranosus & Semitendinosus

Action

Flexes the knee and extends the hip. Internally rotates the tibia in the flexed knee.

The semimembranosus and semitendinosus contract, bending the knee and internally rotating the tibia in Marichyasana I. This internal rotation manifests as external rotation of the hip, accentuating the twist of the trunk.

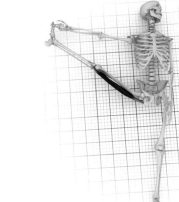

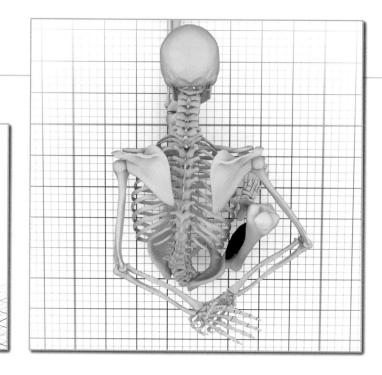

Awakening

The semimembranosus and semitendinosus stretch and awaken in Supta Padangusthasana B.

Hamstrings

Contracted

Iliopsoas lunge: Contracting the hamstrings of the front leg draws the body forward, accentuating the stretch of the iliopsoas in lunging postures.

Stretched

Krounchasana: This Asana stretches all hamstrings. Contracting the iliopsoas on the side of the bent knee tilts the pelvis forward, drawing the origin of the hamstrings away from the insertion. This accentuates the hamstring stretch.

Hamstrings

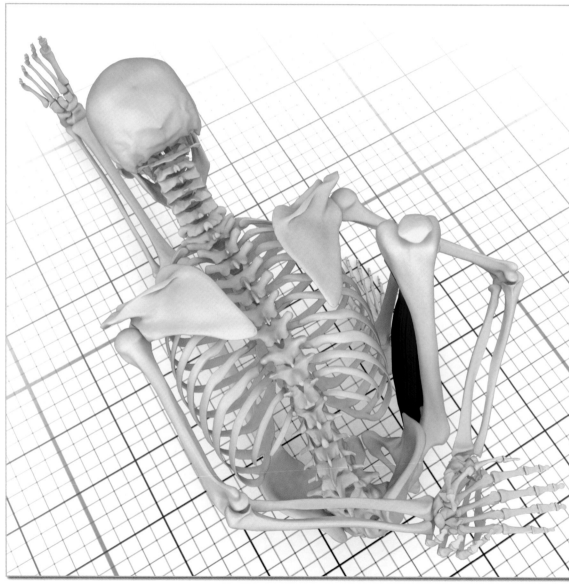

Marichyasana I

The seated twists are named in honor of the great sage Maha Rishi. Their tortional action compresses and expands the internal organs, flushing blood into the veins. The veins have one-way valves that then direct this blood to the heart.

All muscles having rotational action contribute to twists including the rotator cuff, the external rotators of the hip, and the hamstrings.

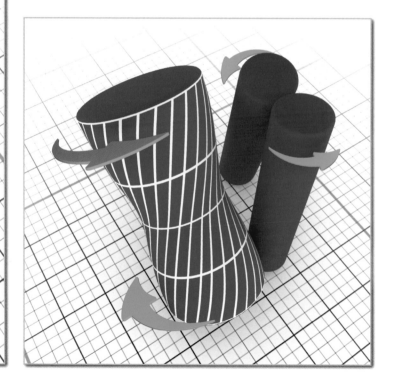

Marichyasana III

Twisting postures awaken the muscles of the trunk, stimulating sensory nerve conduction from the skin, myofacial layers, and the muscles themselves. This illuminates and drives the subtle energies of the Chakras upward though the Sushumna Nadi (spinal cord).

The semimembranosus and semitendinosus contract in Marichyasana I. The biceps femoris contracts in Marichyasana III.

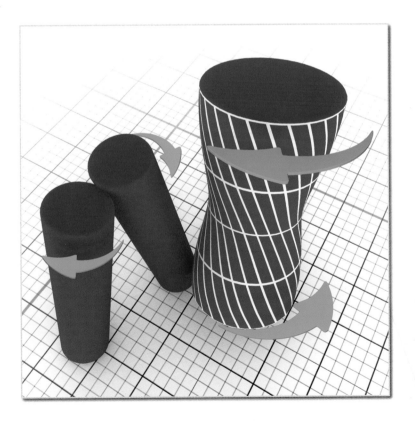

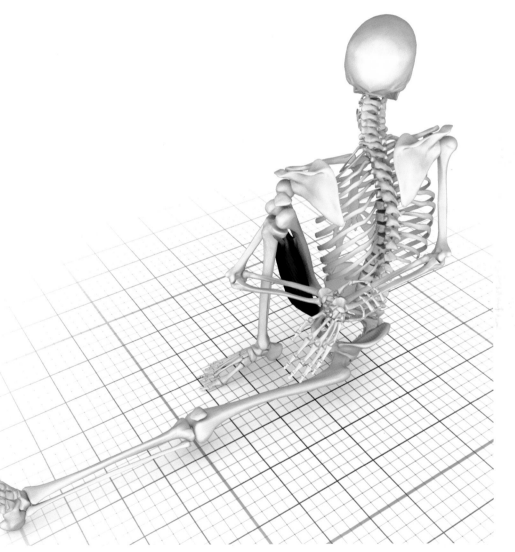

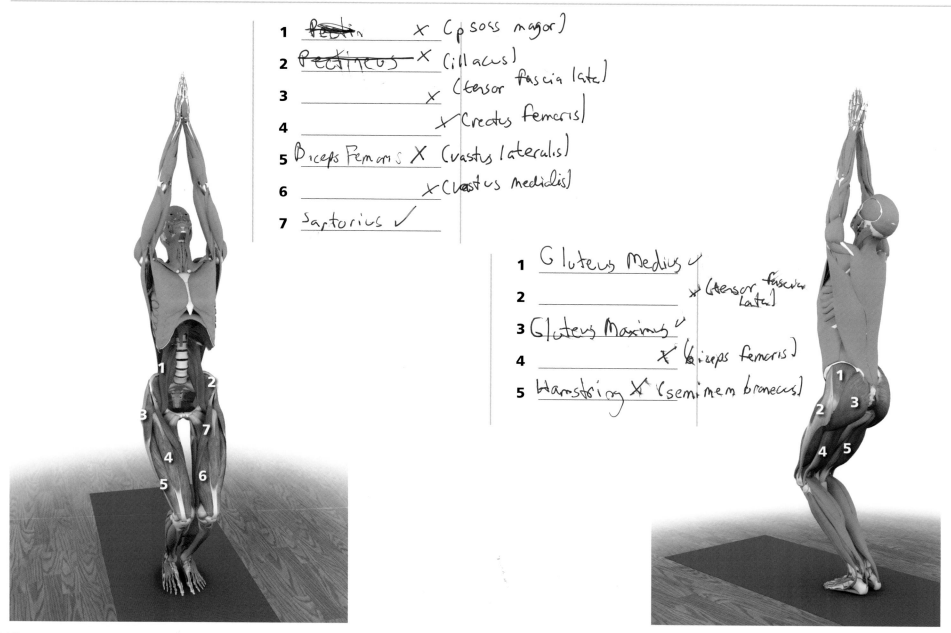

1 ~~Pectin~~ ✗ (psoss major)

2 ~~Pectineus~~ ✗ (iliacus)

3 _____ ✗ (tensor fascia late)

4 _____ ✗ (rectus femoris)

5 Biceps Femoris ✗ (vastus lateralis)

6 _____ ✗ (vastus medialis)

7 Sartorius ✓

1 Gluteus Medius ✓

2 _____ ✗ (tensor fascia lata)

3 Gluteus Maximus ✓

4 _____ ✗ (biceps femoris)

5 Hamstring ✗ (semi membranosus)

Please see www.BandhaYoga.com for answers...

Part Two

The Trunk

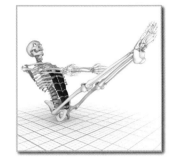
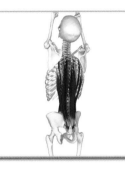
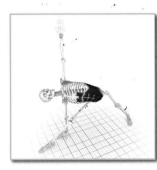
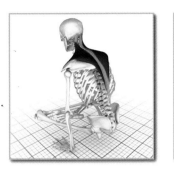
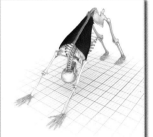
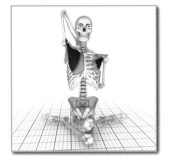

1 pectoralis major

2 external oblique

3 rectus abdominis

4 pectoralis minor

5 intercostals

6 internal oblique

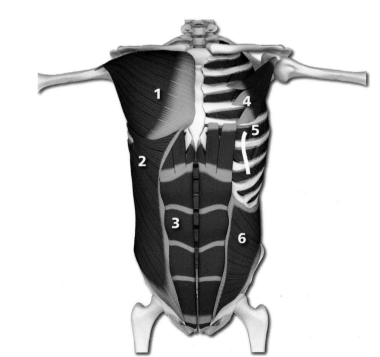

Left to right illustrates the muscles of the back, from deep to superficial

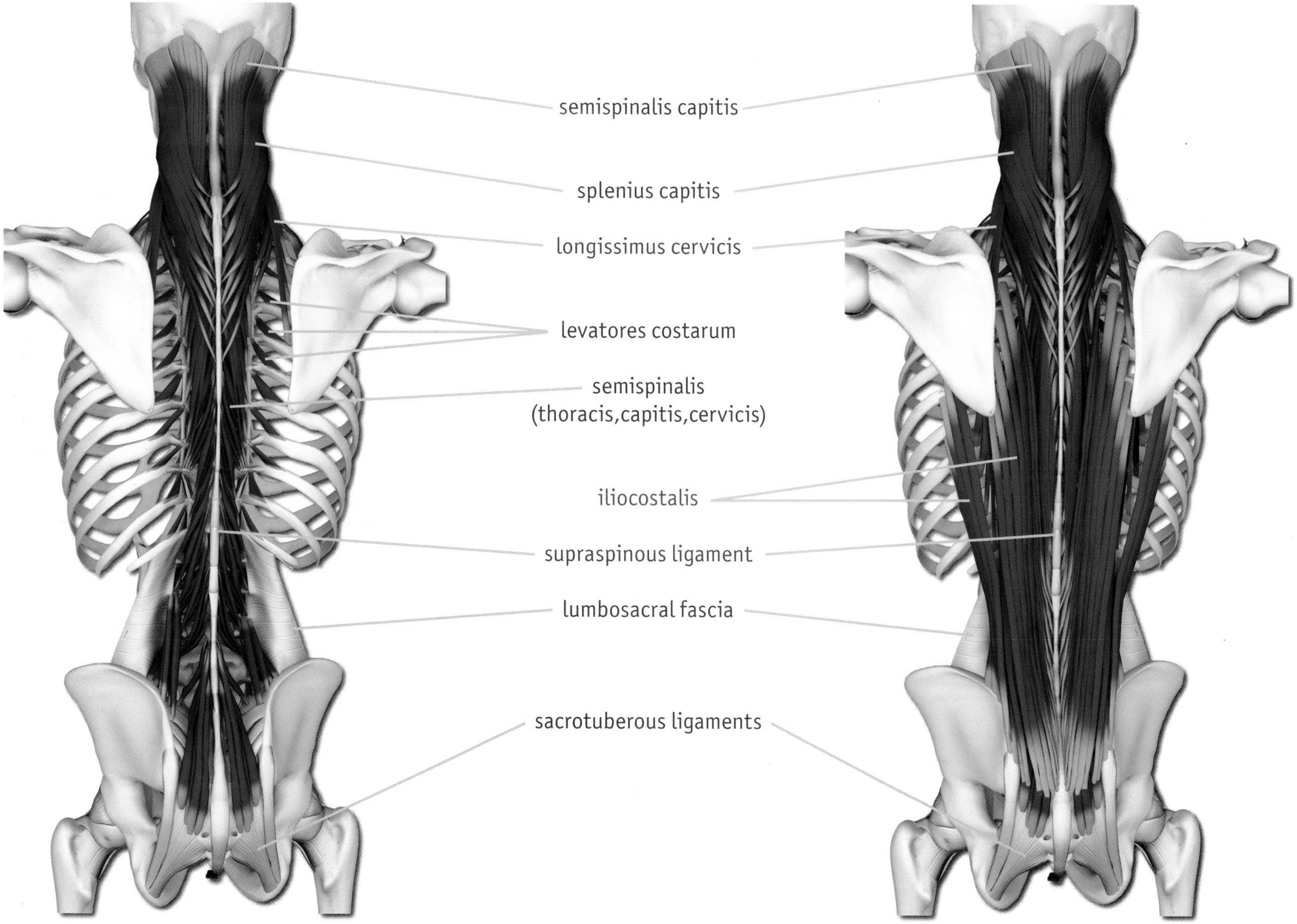

semispinalis capitis

splenius capitis

longissimus cervicis

levatores costarum

semispinalis
(thoracis, capitis, cervicis)

iliocostalis

supraspinous ligament

lumbosacral fascia

sacrotuberous ligaments

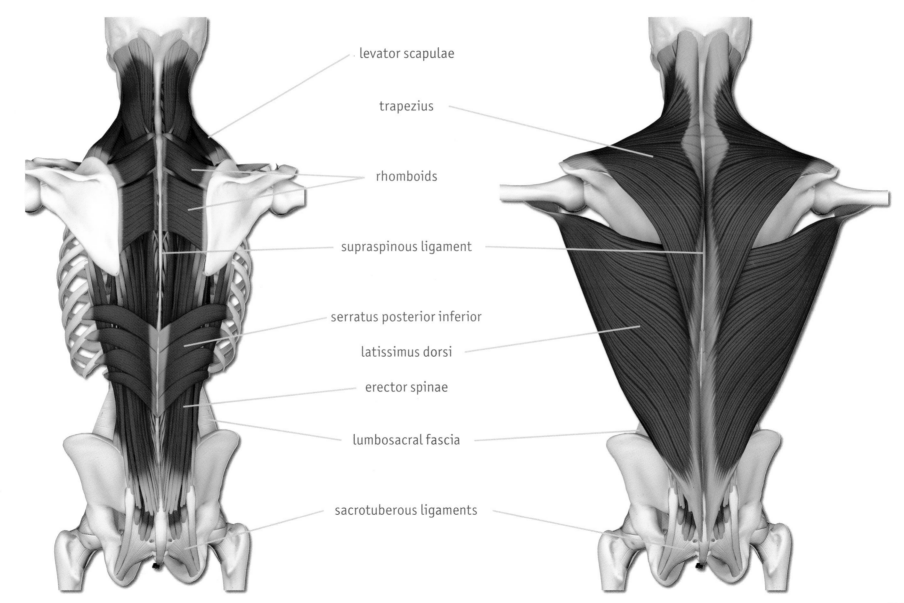

levator scapulae

trapezius

rhomboids

supraspinous ligament

serratus posterior inferior

latissimus dorsi

erector spinae

lumbosacral fascia

sacrotuberous ligaments

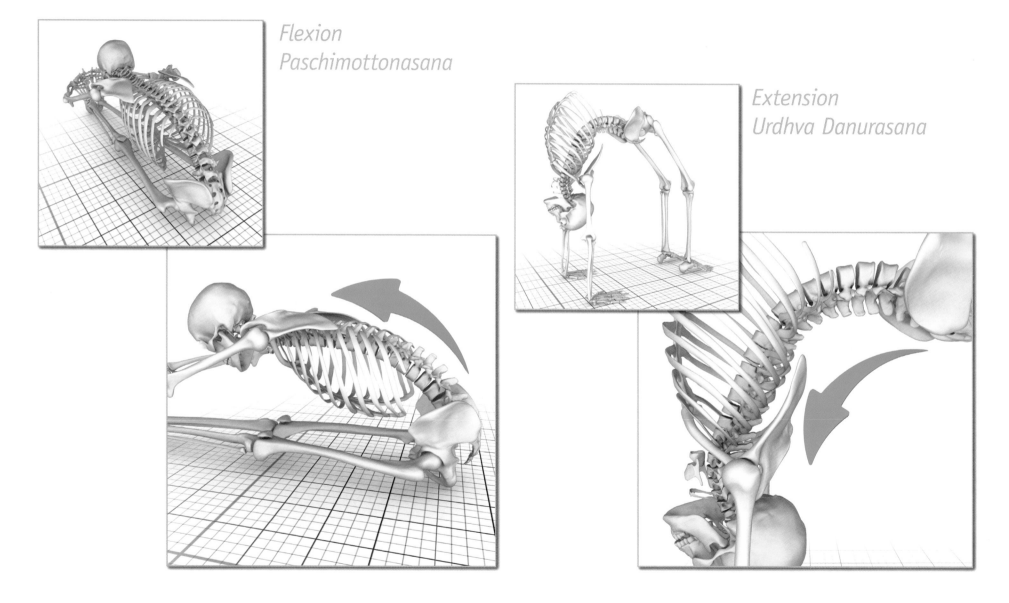

Flexion
Paschimottonasana

Extension
Urdhva Danurasana

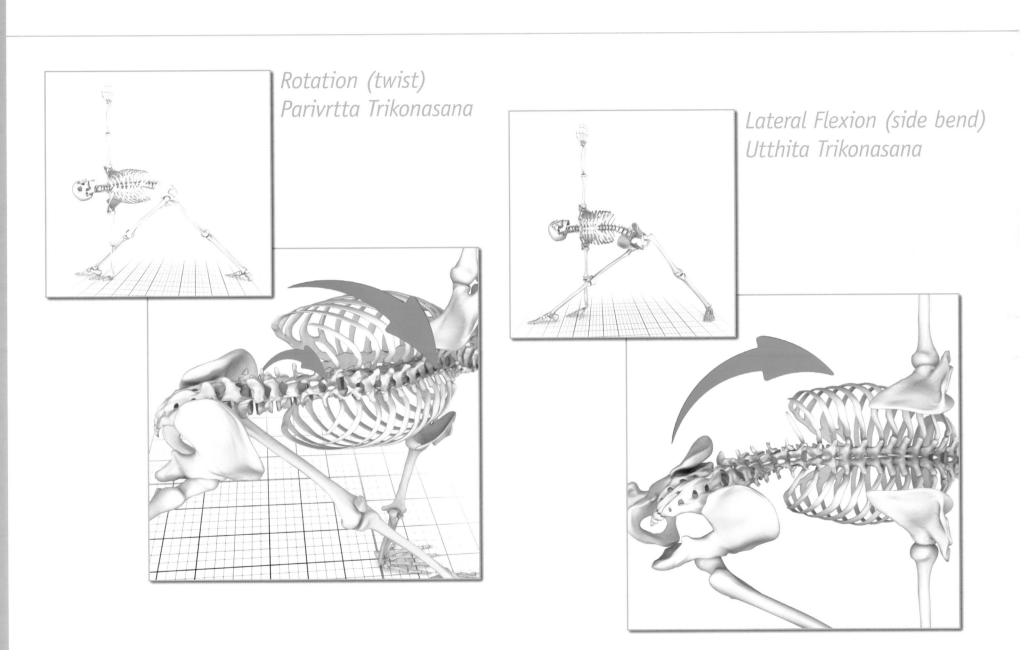

Rotation (twist)
Parivrtta Trikonasana

Lateral Flexion (side bend)
Utthita Trikonasana

Chapter 9

Abdominals

Rectus Abdominis (REK-tus ab-DOM-i-nus)

Internal Oblique (o-BLEEK)

External Oblique (o-BLEEK)

Transversus Abdominis

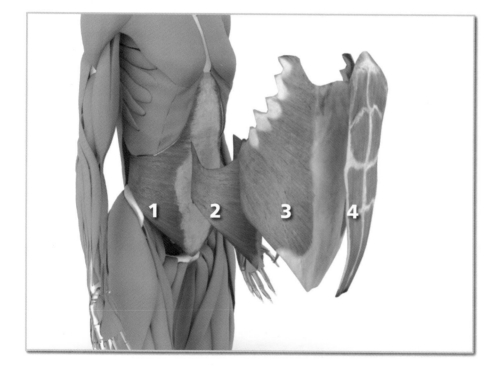

1 Transversus Abdominis

2 Internal Oblique

3 External Oblique

4 Rectus Abdominis

Rectus Abdominis

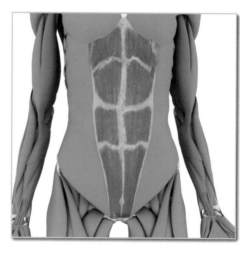

This is a long flat muscle that is divided into four bellies by horizontal fibrous bands, giving it a "washboard" appearance. It originates bilaterally from the pubic symphysis and pubic crest, inserting on the xyphoid process (at the bottom of the sternum) and, more laterally, the cartilage of the fifth, sixth, and seventh ribs.

Contracting the rectus abdominis flexes the trunk forward, or, if the insertion is fixed, lifts the pelvis. This is demonstrated in Uttanasana and Tolasana, respectively. Tightness in this muscle limits the depth of back bends such as Urdhva Danurasana and Purvottanasana.

Contracting the rectus abdominis also compresses the abdominal contents, producing an "air bag" effect, which is thought to prevent hyperextension of the lumbar spine, protecting it when extended (as in back bends).

External Oblique

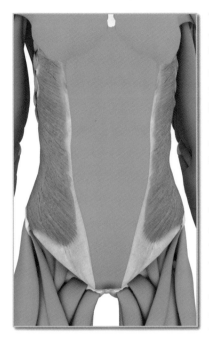

This is a sheet-like muscle with fibers running opposite to the internal oblique. It is the larger of the two obliques and lies superficial. Its anterior fibers are more superior, originating from the front of the ribs, crossing diagonally forward and downward, and inserting on the linea alba. Its lateral fibers are more posterior, originating from the back of the ribs, crossing downward and forward, and inserting on the structures at the front of the pelvis.

Contraction of the external oblique draws the shoulder forward. This action combines with contraction of the contralateral (other side) internal oblique, accentuating twisting poses. Tightness in this muscle limits these postures. Contraction assists in compressing the abdominal contents and contributes to the "air bag" effect, protecting the lumbar spine.

Internal Oblique

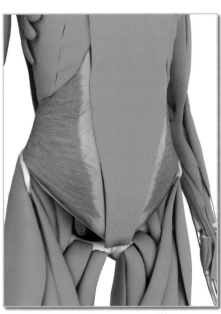

This is a thin sheet-like muscle located on the side of the trunk. Its fibers cross diagonally upward and forward from the iliac crest, inserting on the lower ribs and the linea alba (a band of fibrous tissue running down the front of the abdomen).

Contraction of the internal oblique draws the opposite shoulder forward and bends the trunk laterally. This action accentuates twisting postures such as Parivrtta Trikonasana. Contracting the internal oblique also contributes to the "air bag" effect described for the rectus abdominis.

Transversus Abdominis

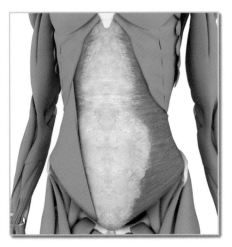

The transversus abdominis is the deepest of the abdominal muscles. Its fibers run horizontally, originating on the iliac crest, the inguinal ligament, and the thoracolumbar fascia and inserting on the lower costal cartilages. Contracting the transversus abdominis compresses the abdomen and tones the abdominal organs. This muscle is important for Udyana Bandha and Nali. Awaken and strengthen it in Navasana.

Abdominals

Origin-Rectus Abdominis

Symphysis pubis and pubic crest.

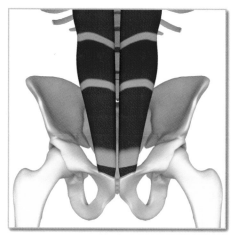

Origin-Internal Oblique

Lower borders of the lateral third of the inguinal ligament, iliac crest, thoracolumbar fascia, and linea alba.

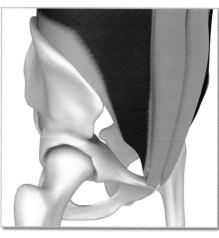

Origin-External Oblique

Ribs 5 through 12 and lower section of the latissimus dorsi.

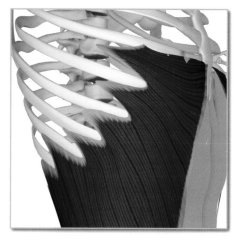

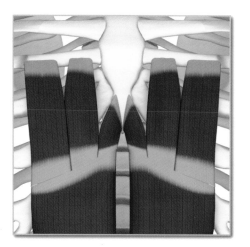

Insertion-Rectus Abdominis

Zyphoid process, costal cartilages 5, 6, and 7.

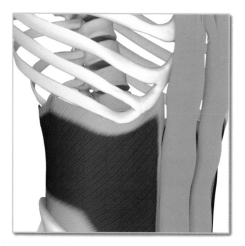

Insertion-Internal Oblique

Linea alba and ribs 9 through 12.

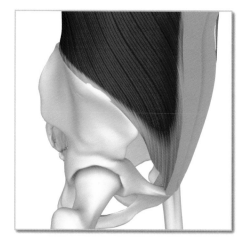

Insertion-External Oblique

Linea alba, inguinal ligament, and anterior half of the iliac crest.

Transversus Abdominis Origin and Insertion

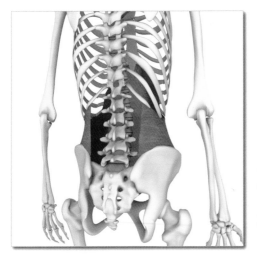

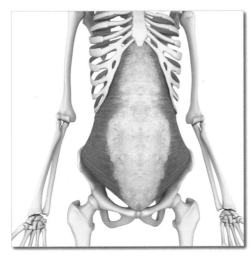

Origin: Iliac crest, inguinal ligament, and thoracolumbar fascia.

Insertion: Lower costal cartilages.

Innervation & Chakra Illuminated

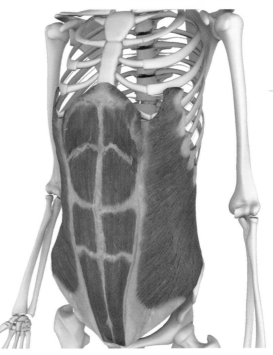

Intercostal nerves (thoracic nerves 7 through 12), iliohypogastric and ilioinguinal nerves (thoracic nerve 12 and lumbar nerve 1).

Chakra illuminated: Third.

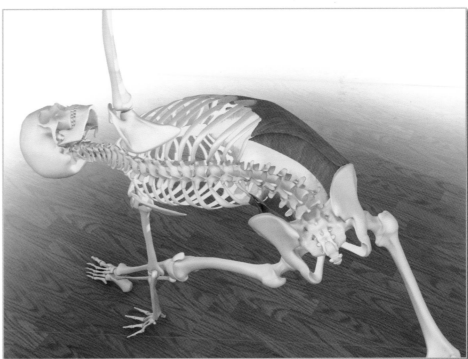

Abdominals

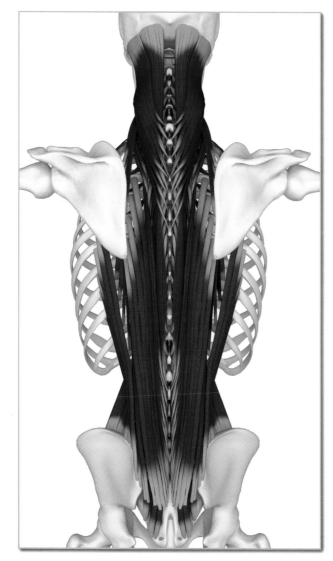

Abdominals–Antagonists

Erector spinae and quadratus lumborum.

Obliques–Antagonists

Same-side muscles are rotational antagonists.

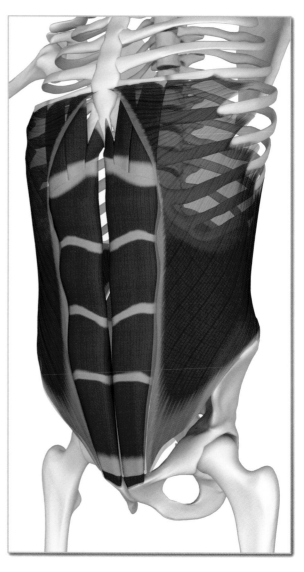

Abdominals–Synergists

Each other (for abdominal compression).

Obliques–Synergists

Opposite-side muscles are rotational synergists. They can assist each other, turning the body.

Rectus Abdominis

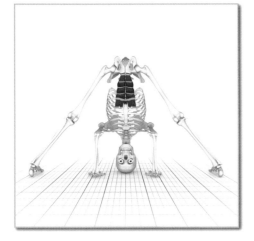

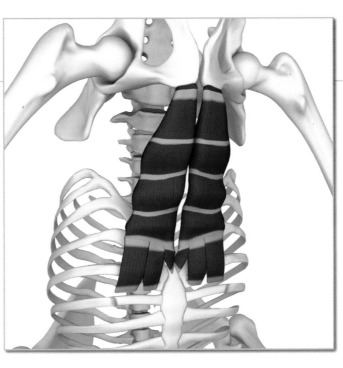

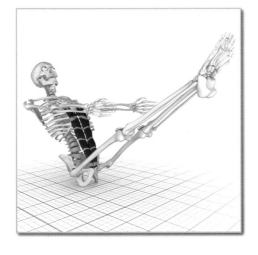

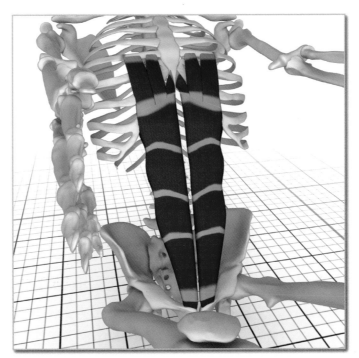

Action

Flexes the trunk and compresses the abdomen.

Contracting the rectus abdominis draws the trunk forward and deepens Prasarita Padottanasana. Contracting the iliopsoas and quadriceps accentuates this action.

Awakening

The rectus abdominis awakens in Navasana.

Obliques

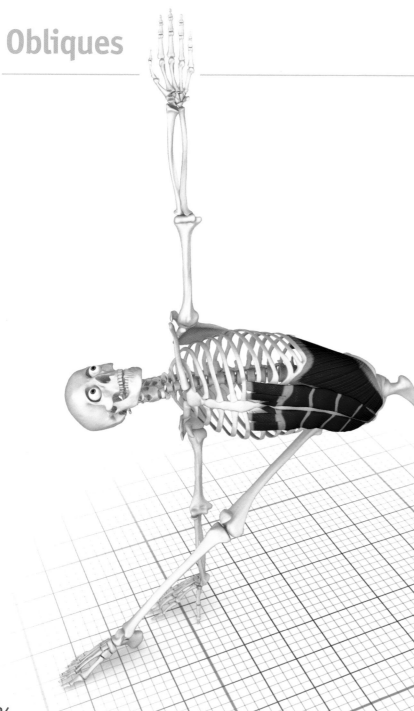

Action and Awakening

1) External Oblique: Unilateral (one-sided) contraction rotates the same-side shoulder forward and laterally flexes the trunk.

Bilateral contraction flexes the trunk and compresses the abdomen.

2) Internal Oblique: Unilateral contraction rotates the contralateral (opposite side) shoulder forward and laterally flexes the trunk.

Bilateral contraction flexes the trunk and compresses the abdomen.

The upper-side internal oblique and the lower-side external oblique contract in Utthita Trikonasana, turning the trunk. Their opposites are lengthened by this action.

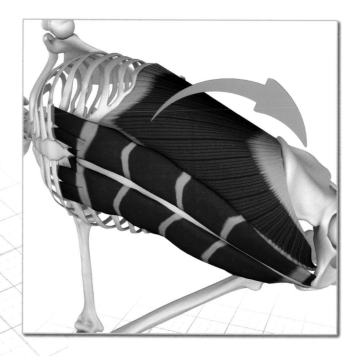

Abdominals

The "Airbag" Effect

Contracting the abdominal muscles compresses the abdominal organs and provides additional support to the muscles surrounding the lumbar spine. This mechanism comes into play when we lift a heavy object and in "valsalva." This concept can be applied during Yoga postures. Only light contraction is necessary to benefit from this action.

Light contraction of the abdominals in back bends also opposes hyperextension of the lumbar spine and tones the abdominals (through eccentric contraction). Contracting the abdominals in this way activates Udyana Bandha (in the region of the solar plexus), illuminating the third Chakra.

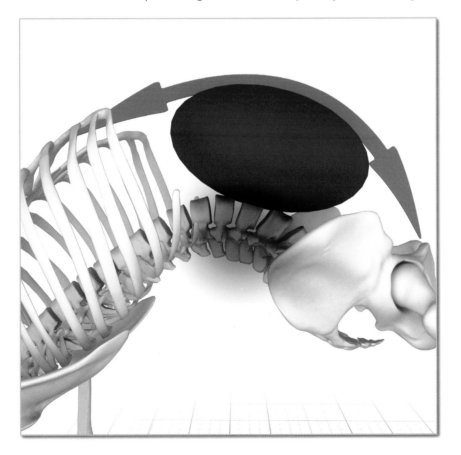

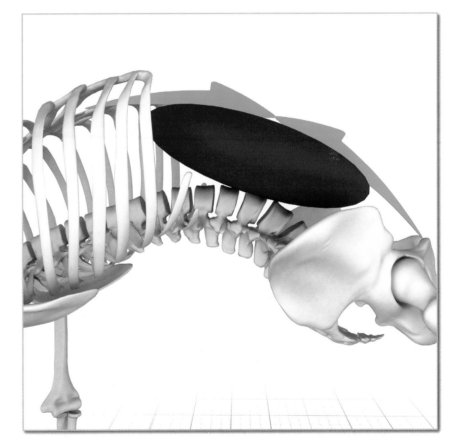

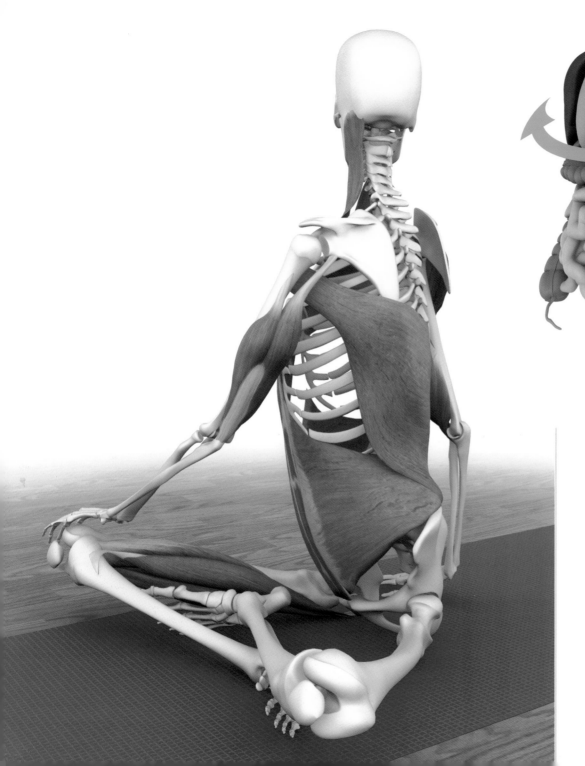

Twisting and Detoxification

Twisting postures create a "wringing" effect on the abdominal organs. This helps to flush the liver and other organs, directing blood and lymphatic fluid into the larger vessels of the cardiovascular system, eliminating toxins.

The abdominal muscles are the core prime movers in the twisting postures. Combine them with other muscular synergists of the twist. For example, in twisting Siddhasana, the sternocleidomastoid, latissimus dorsi, and triceps of one side assist the biceps and hamstrings of the other side to accentuate the twist.

Synergy

Combine the actions of various muscles to create synergy in your posture. Contract the posture's synergists to lengthen the antagonists.

These illustrations demonstrate that contracting the rectus abdominis, iliopsoas, quadriceps, deltoids, and biceps in Prasarita Padottanasana stretch the erector spinae, hamstring, and gastrocnemius muscles.

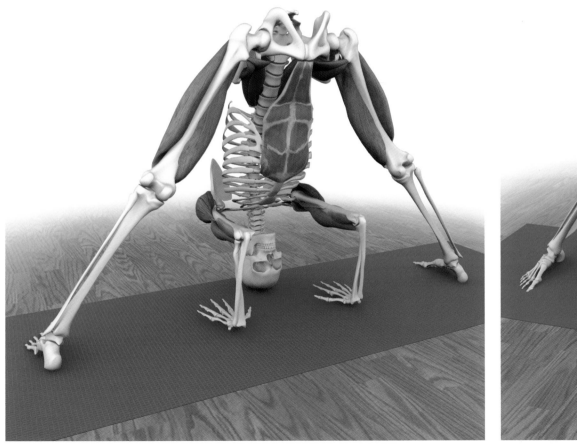

Prasarita Padotanasana–synergists

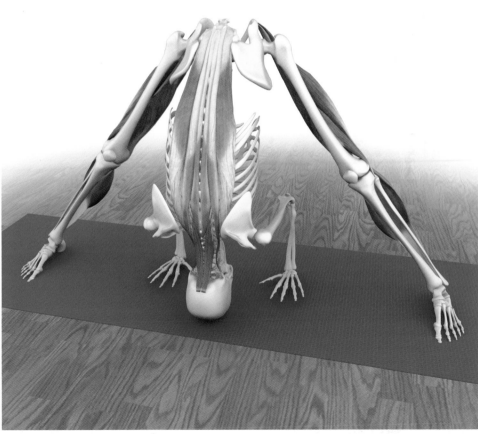

Prasarita Padotanasana–antagonists

Chapter 10

Back Muscles

Erector Spinae
(EE-rec-tor SPEE-neh)

This group has three sets of muscles running parallel to the vertebral column. The spinalis runs up the center of the back from one vertebral spinous process to the next. The longissimus muscles are more lateral and run from the ilium to the vertebral transverse processes and the ribs. The iliocostalis are the most lateral and run from one rib to the next. Contracting these muscles straightens the spine, as in Tadasana. Contracting the laterally placed longissimus and iliocostalis produces lateral bending, as in Utthita Trikonasana. Contracting one side or the other produces a rotational effect in twisting postures.

Forward bends such as Uttanasana and Kurmasana stretch these muscles. When they reach full length, they tilt the pelvis forward by pulling on the back of the ilium. This tilt draws the ischial tuberosity upward and stretches the hamstrings. Back bends such as Urdhva Danurasana strengthen these muscles.

Quadratus Lumborum
(quad-RA-tus lum-BOR-um)

Deep to the erector spinae lies the quadratus lumborum, a combination of five heads that form a square-shaped muscle. They have a common origin from the posterior iliac crest, dividing into four parts, inserting on the transverse processes of the lumbar vertebrae and the posterior section of rib 12. Contracting the quadratus lumborum unilaterally flexes the trunk to the side in Utthita Trikonasana. Contracting both sides extends the lumbar spine in Urdhva Danurasana.

When the pelvis is fixed, contracting the quadratus lumborum draws the ribcage downward. This action can be used to deepen respiration.

The quadratus lumborum and psoas major wrap around the lumbar spine and stabilize it. Contracting the quadratus lumborum, psoas major, and rectus abdominis protects the lumbar spine in back bends.

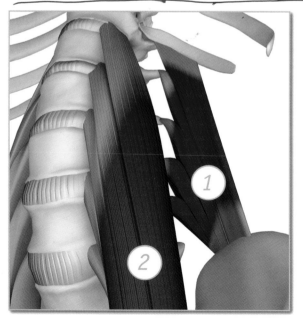

1) Quadratus Lumborum
2) Psoas Major

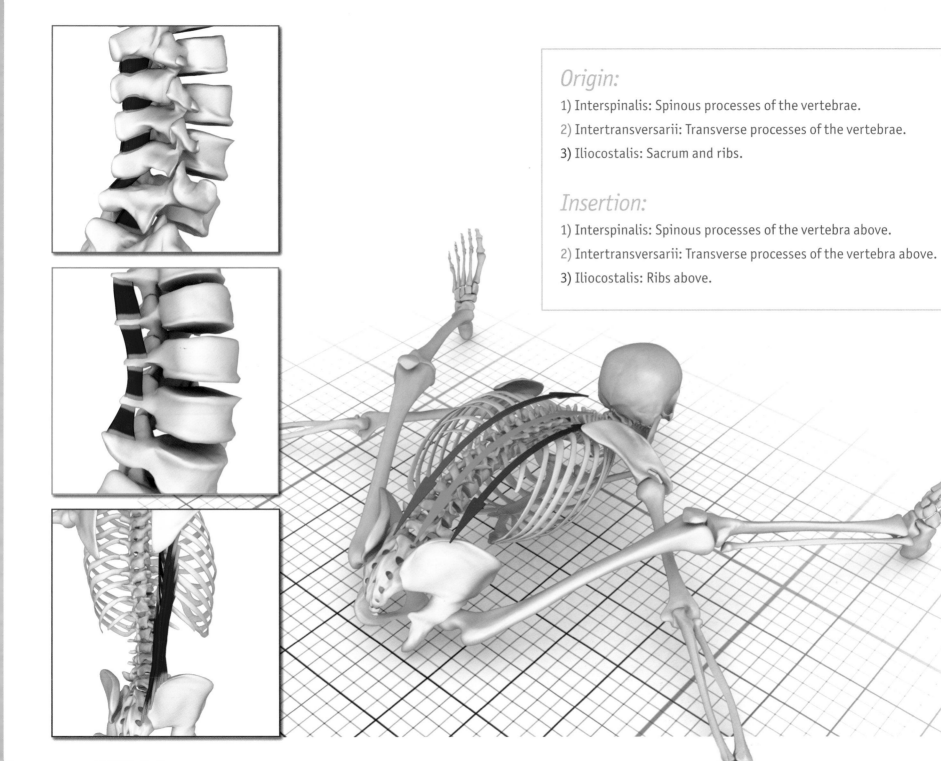

Origin:

1) Interspinalis: Spinous processes of the vertebrae.

2) Intertransversarii: Transverse processes of the vertebrae.

3) Iliocostalis: Sacrum and ribs.

Insertion:

1) Interspinalis: Spinous processes of the vertebra above.

2) Intertransversarii: Transverse processes of the vertebra above.

3) Iliocostalis: Ribs above.

Back Muscles

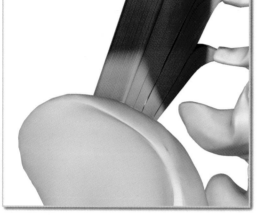

Lower thoracic and upper lumbar nerves.

Chakra illuminated: Third and fourth.

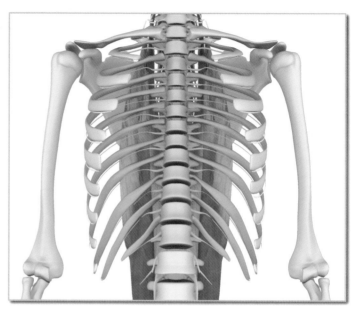

Origin
Quadratus Lumborum

Medial iliac crest.

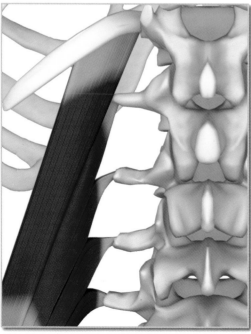

Insertion
Quadratus Lumborum

Lower border of rib 12 and the transverse processes of lumbar vertebrae 1 through 4.

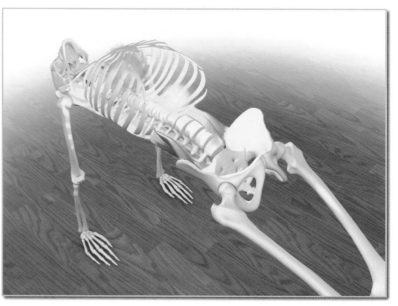

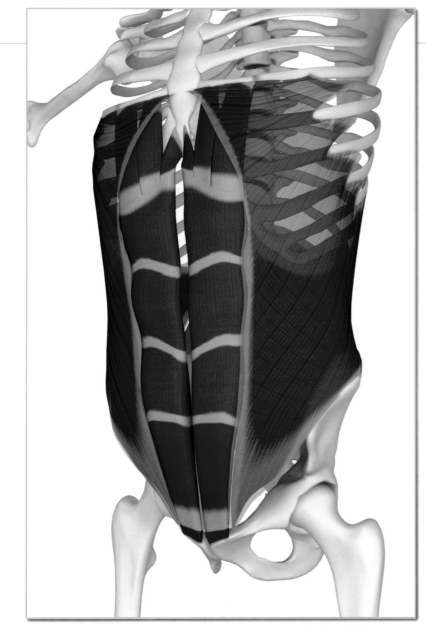

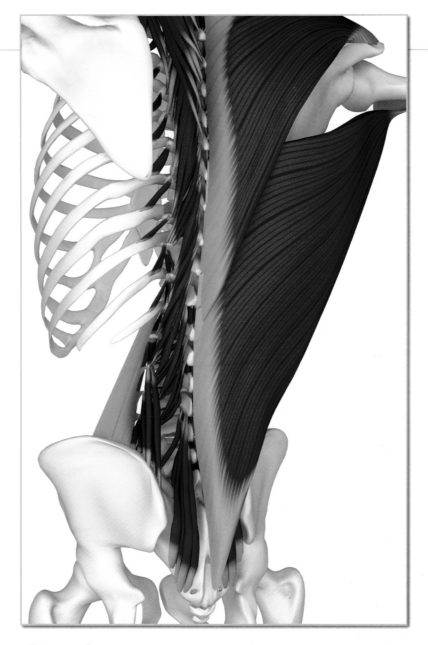

Abdominals.

Each other, latissimus dorsi, trapezius.

Back Muscles

Action

Extends, laterally flexes, and assists in rotating the vertebral column.

The laterally placed erector spinae and the deeper quadratus lumborum contract to twist the back and lift the kidney region in poses such as Marichyasana III.

The erector spinae and quadratus lumborum lift and straighten the spine in Tadasana.

Open-chain contraction of the quadratus lumborum draws the ribs downward during respiration.

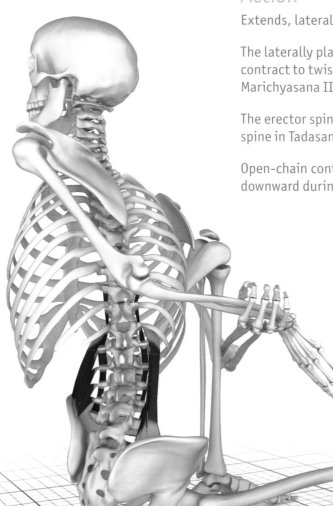

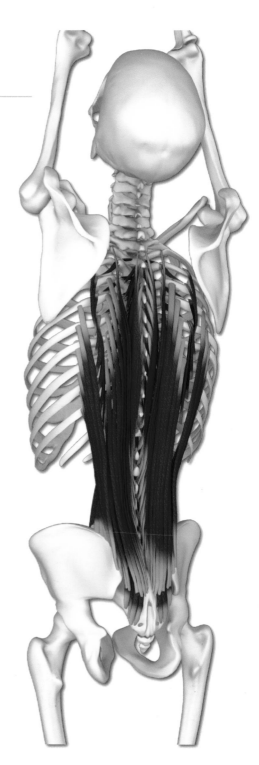

Synergy

The erector spinae muscles are the prime movers in the back bend Purvottanasana. Combine contraction of the erector spinae with the synergists of this pose, including the quadriceps, gluteus maximus, and triceps. This combination stretches the rectus femoris, iliopsoas, rectus abdominis, pectoralis major, biceps, and anterior neck muscles.

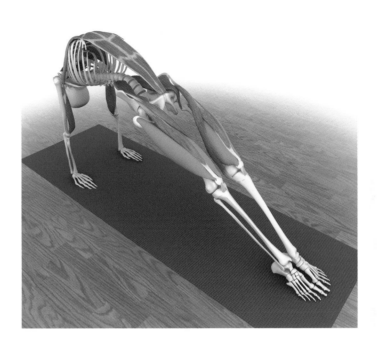

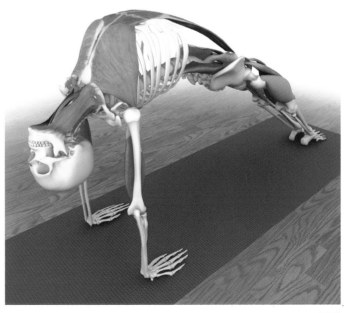

Purvottanasana

Chapter 11

Latissimus Dorsi

The latissimus dorsi forms two-thirds of the superficial back muscles, originating from the posterior iliac crest, sacrum, and thoracolumbar fascia, rotating 180° before inserting on the inside of the proximal humerus. This "twist" increases the torque generated by contraction of the latissimus dorsi. This muscle draws the arm down and toward the body from the overhead position, internally rotating the humerus. When the humerus is fixed (as in certain twists or in Upward Dog), contraction of the latissimus draws the chest forward and opens it. Tightness limits overhead postures such as Virabhadrasana I, Urdhva Danurasana, and Adho Mukha Svanasana.

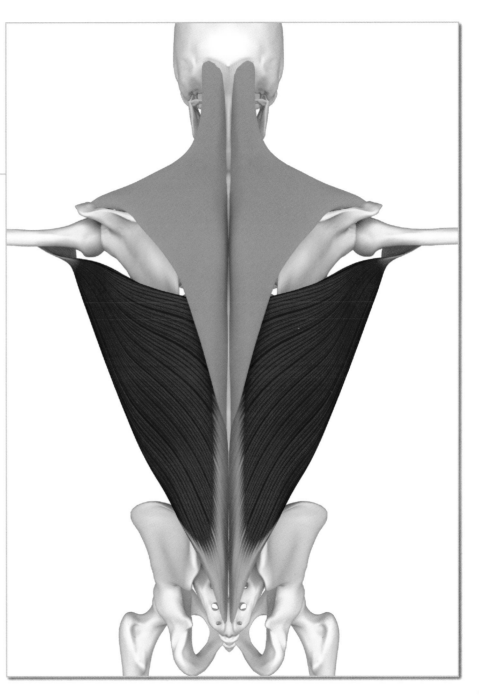

Latissimus Dorsi (luh-TIS-uh-mus DOR-si)

Origin *(back view)*

The iliac crest, thoracolumbar fascia, spinous processes of sacral vertebrae 1 through 5, lumbar vertebrae 1 through 5, thoracic vertebrae 7 through 12, lower 3 ribs, and inferior angle of scapula.

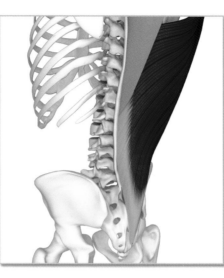

Insertion *(front view)*

Floor of the bicipital groove of the humerus.

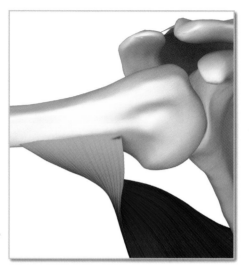

Innervation & Chakra Illuminated

Thoracodorsal nerve (cervical nerves 6, 7, and 8).

Chakra illuminated: Fourth.

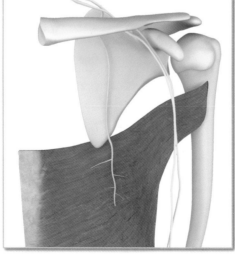

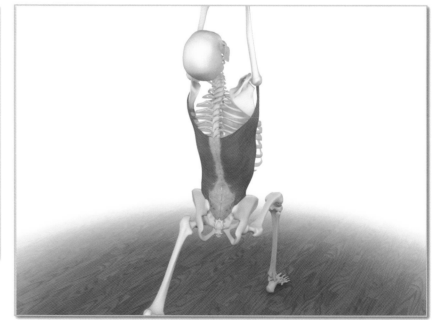

Antagonists

Anterior deltoids, pectoralis major (clavicular portion), and long head of the biceps.

Synergists

Posterior deltoids and pectoralis major (sternocostal portion extends the humerus). Long head of the triceps.

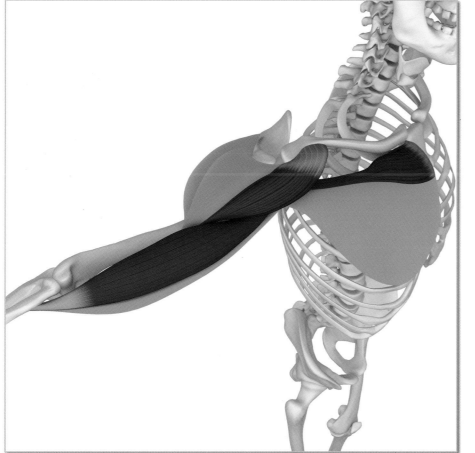

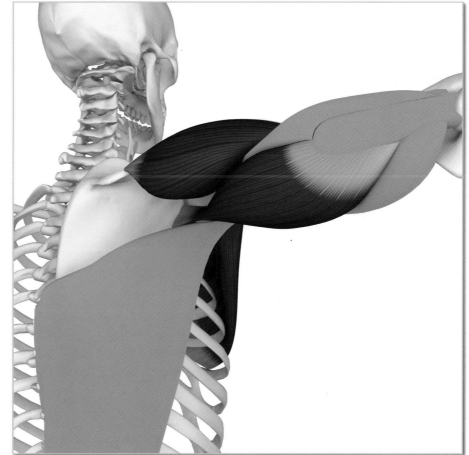

Latissimus Dorsi (luh-TIS-uh-mus DOR-si)

Action

Extends the arm (from a flexed position). Internally rotates and adducts the arm.

The latissimus dorsi contract, drawing the lower back upward and opening the chest in Urdhva Mukha Svanasana.

Awakening

The latissimus dorsi stretches in Adho Mukha Svanasana.

The latissimus dorsi, in association with the pectoralis major, draws the body forward and through the arms during the transition from Adho Mukha Svanasana to Urdhva Mukha Svanasana.

Chapter 12

Trapezius

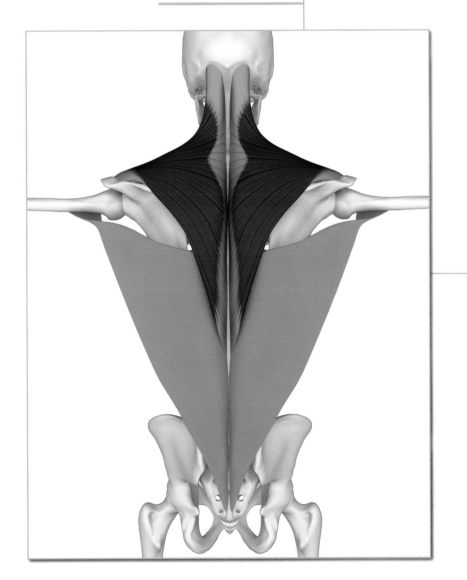

This is a broad triangular-shaped muscle originating from the center of the back, extending from the lower thoracic spine to the base of the skull, and inserting on the scapula and clavicle. Contraction of the lower fibers draws the scapula downward. Contraction of the upper fibers elevates and rotates the scapula upward. This action increases contact of the humeral head with the glenoid in overhead movements (such as full arm balance). Contraction of the middle fibers adducts the scapula, assisting the rhomboids in opening the chest.

Tightness in the middle fibers limits postures such as Gomukhasana B. Weakness in the lower and upper fibers limits arm balances such as Tolasana and Vrksasana, respectively.

Trapezius (tra-PE-ze-us)

Origin

Base of the skull, posterior ligaments of the neck, and spinous processes of cervical vertebra 2 through thoracic vertebra 12.

(The illustration shows upper, middle, and lower fibers of the trapezius.)

Innervation & Chakra Illuminated

Accessory nerve (cranial nerve 11 and cervical nerves 3 and 4).

Chakra illuminated: Fifth.

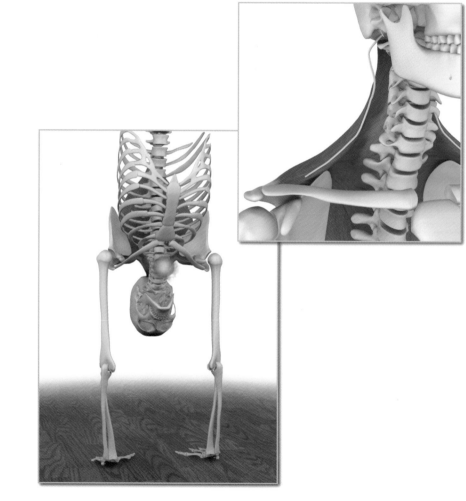

Insertion (top view)

Posterior aspect of the lateral third of the clavicle, medial margin of the acromion, and superior spine of the scapula.

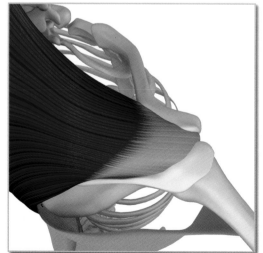

Antagonists Lower Fibers

Upper fibers of trapezius, rhomboid major, rhomboid minor, and sternocleidomastoid.

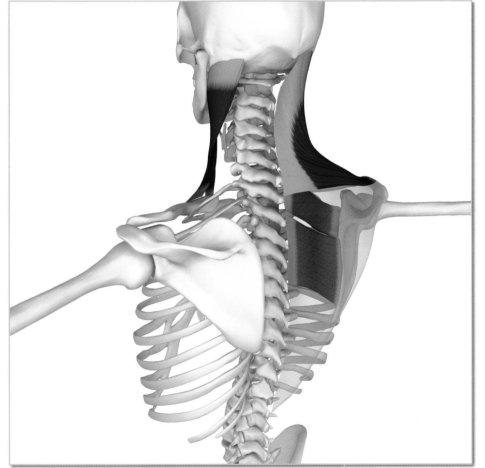

Antagonists Upper Fibers

Lower fibers of trapezius, pectoralis minor, pectoralis major, and latissimus dorsi.

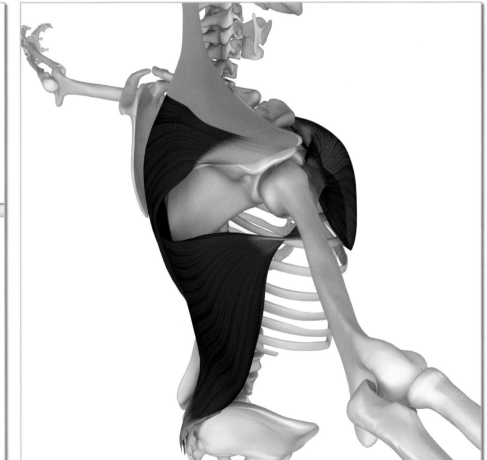

Trapezius (tra-PE-ze-us)

Synergists–Lower Fibers

Pectoralis minor and major and latissimus dorsi.

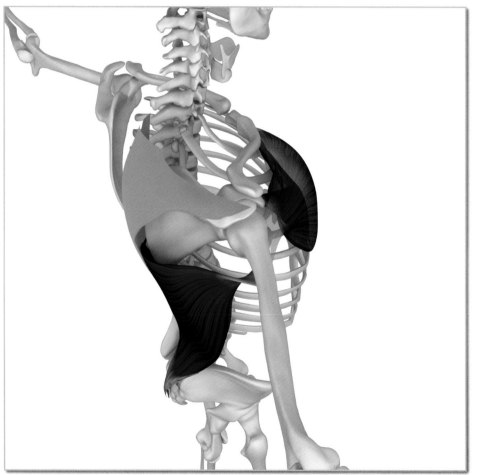

Synergists–Upper Fibers

Anterior and lateral deltoids, rhomboids major and minor, and sternocleidomastoid.

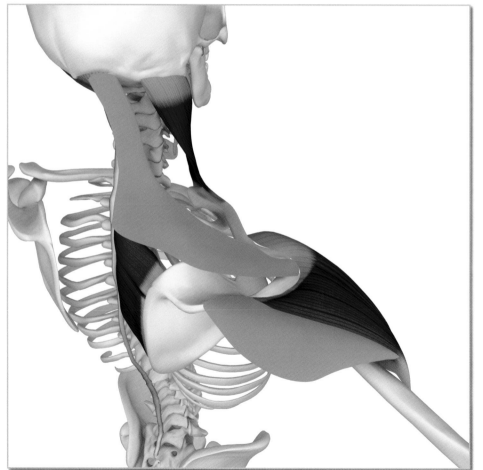

Action

The upper fibers of the trapezius contract in Urdhva Danurasana, assisting the lift of the upper body, outwardly rotating the scapula, and drawing the glenoid into greater contact with the humeral head.

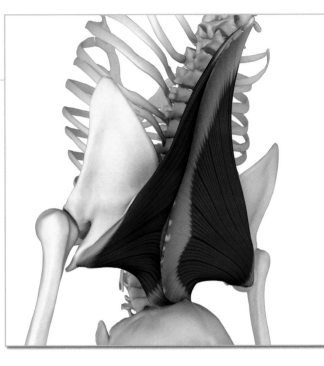

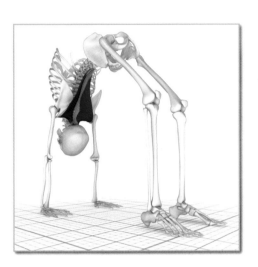

Awakening

The middle and lower fibers of the trapezius contract in Tolasana, lifting the body and retracting the scapulae inward and downward. Weakness in this muscle limits the ability to perform this pose.

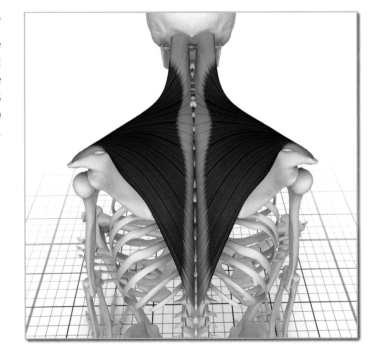

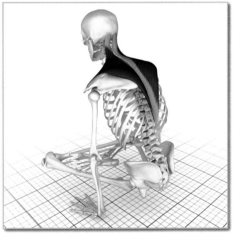

143

Chapter 13

Pectoralis Major & Minor

Pectoralis Minor (pek-to-RA-lis):

This is a small three-headed muscle lying deep to the pectoralis major, originating from the third, fourth, and fifth ribs and inserting on the coracoid process of the scapula. The pectoralis minor draws the scapula downward and forward in open-chain movements.

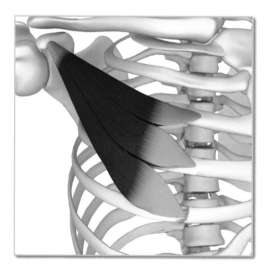

Closed-chain contraction of the pectoralis minor, while stabilizing the scapula posteriorly (with the rhomboids), lifts the ribcage in respiration.

Pectoralis Major

The pectoralis major presents as a large flat muscle forming the front of the chest. The larger sternocostal portion originates from the body of the sternum; the smaller clavicular portion originates from the medial clavicle. Both portions combine to form one tendon, inserting on the inside of the proximal humerus.

Sequential closed-chain contraction of the pectoralis major draws the body forward (as when moving from Downward Dog to Upward Dog). Both portions adduct the humerus (as in Gomukhasana B). This is also a key muscle in push-up poses, such as Chataranga Dandasana. The sternocostal portion stretches in overhead postures, such as Urdhva Danurasana, and tightness limits the depth of these poses.

Origin
Pectoralis Major

Medial third of the clavicle, anterior aspect of the sternum, upper 6 costal cartilages, and aponeurosis of the external oblique.

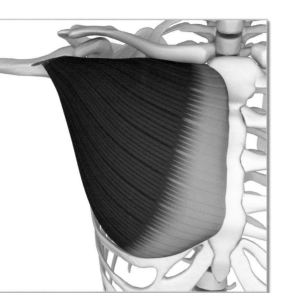

Insertion
Pectoralis Major

Lateral lip of bicipital groove (sternal fibers, more proximally, clavicular fibers insert more distally).

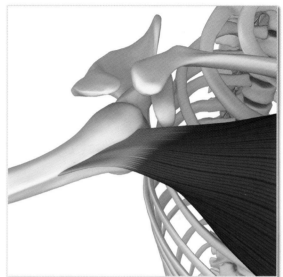

Origin
Pectoralis Minor

Outer surface of ribs 2 through 5.

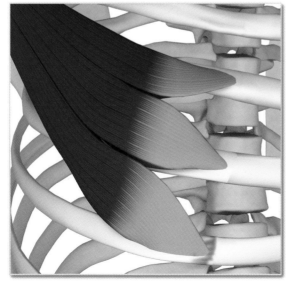

Insertion
Pectoralis Minor

Coracoid process of the scapula.

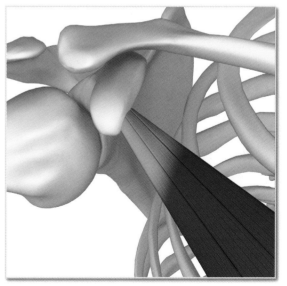

Pectoralis Major & Minor

Antagonists
Pectoralis Major

Middle deltoid, supraspinatus, infraspinatus, and biceps (long head).

Synergists
Pectoralis Major

Latissimus dorsi and triceps (long head).

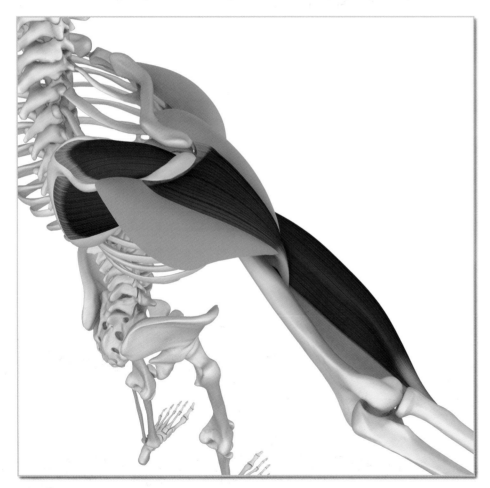

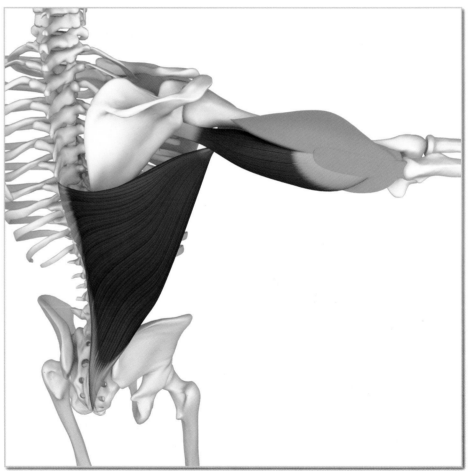

Antagonists
Pectoralis Minor

Sternocleidomastoid and upper fibers of the trapezius.

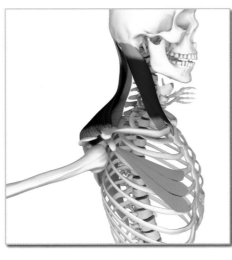

Synergists
Pectoralis Minor

Rhomboid major, rhomboid minor, and latissimus dorsi.

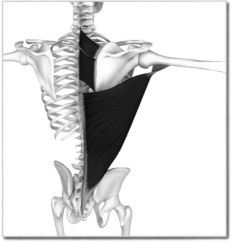

Innervation & Chakra Illuminated

Pectoralis Major:

Clavicular portion: Lateral pectoral nerve (cervical nerves 5 through 7). Sternal portion: Medial pectoral nerve (cervical nerves 8 through thoracic nerve 1).

Pectoralis Minor:

Medial pectoral nerve (cervical nerves 8 through thoracic nerve 1).

Chakra illuminated: Fifth.

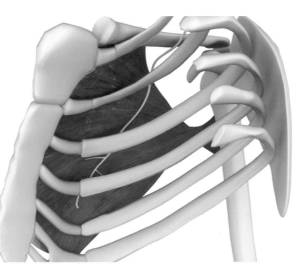

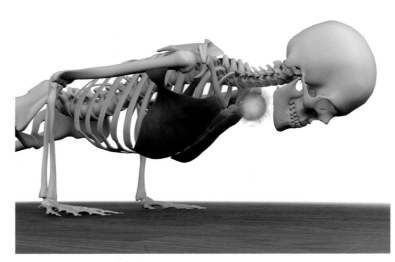

Pectoralis Major & Minor

Action

Adducts and internally rotates the arm.

Flexes the arm from an extended position.

Depresses the arm and shoulder.

The pectoralis major and minor are stretched and awakened in Purvottanasana.

Awakening

Chataranga Dandasana: The pectoralis major and minor (in association with the serratus anterior) stabilize the upper body in this pose.

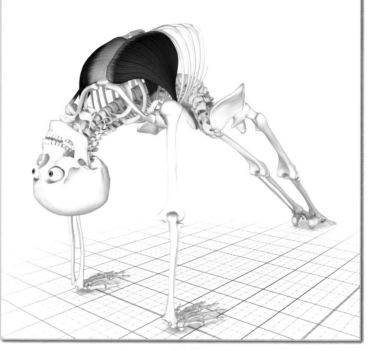

Stretched and Contracted

The upper arm stretches the lower fibers of the pectoralis major. The pectoralis minor contracts, drawing the scapula of the lower arm forward. The rhomboids of the lower arm contract to stabilize the scapula, lifting the ribcage. Eccentrically contracting the upper arm pectoralis major facilitates this stretch (seen here in Gomukhasana B).

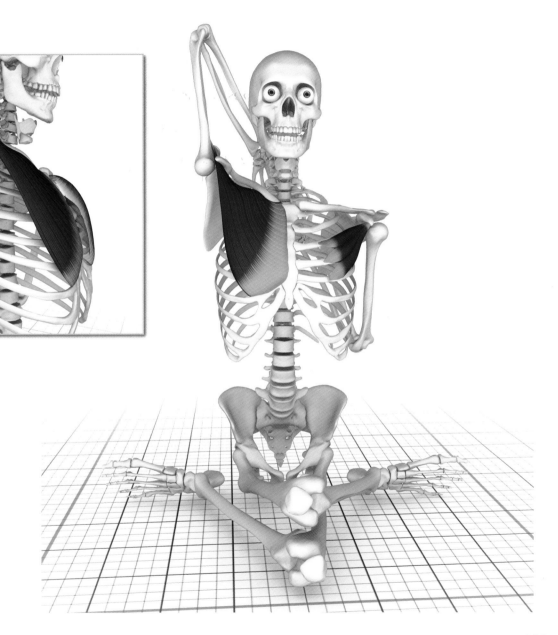

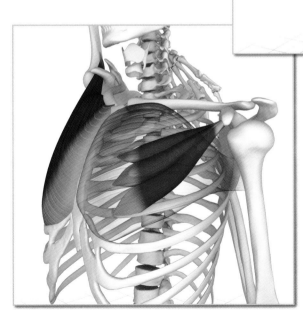

1 Trapezius
2 Pectoralis Major
3 rectust abdominis
4 external oblique

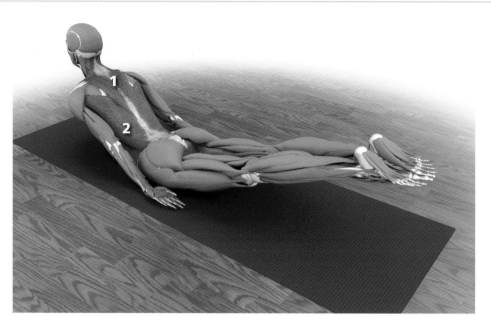

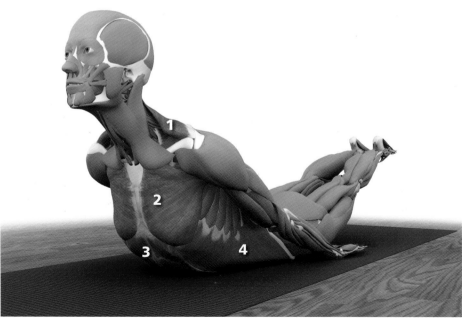

1 Trapezius
2 Latissimus dorsi

Part Three

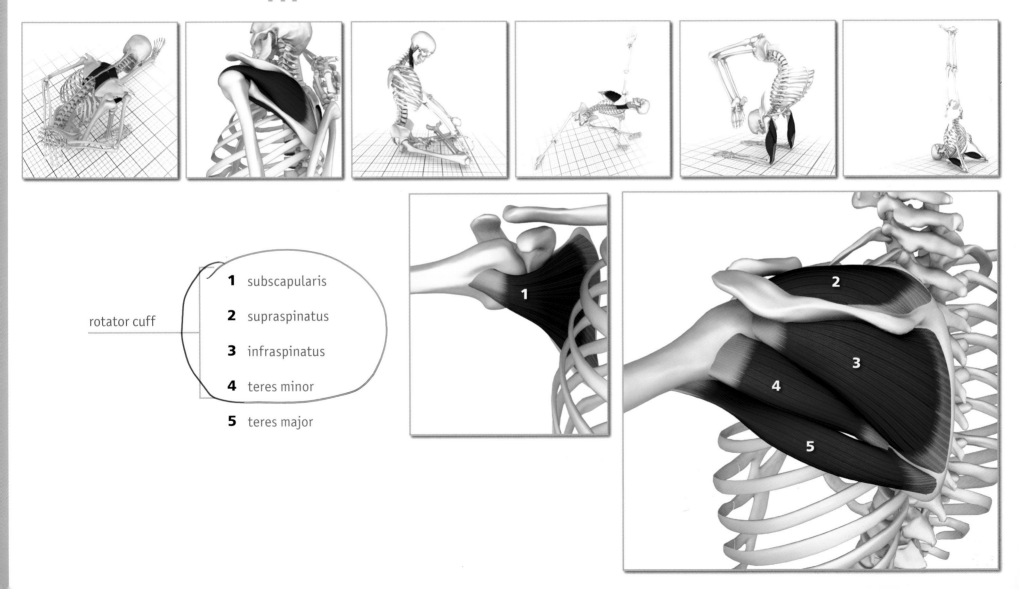

rotator cuff

1 subscapularis

2 supraspinatus

3 infraspinatus

4 teres minor

5 teres major

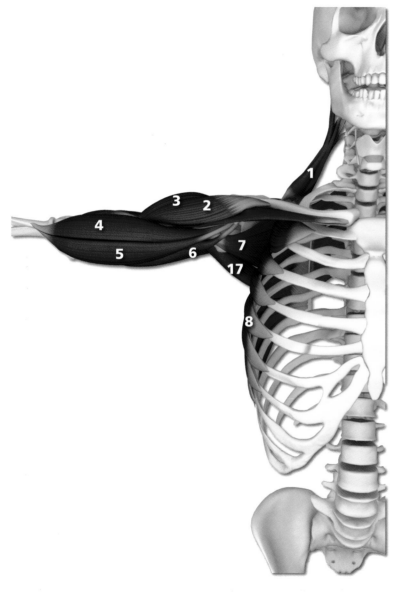

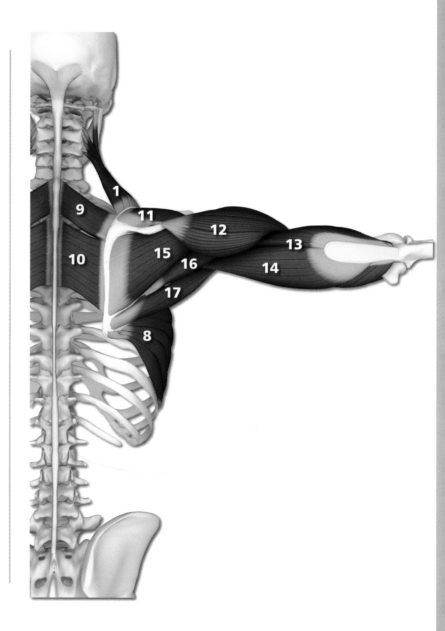

1. levator scapulae
2. anterior deltoid
3. lateral deltoid
4. biceps (long head)
5. biceps (short head)
6. coracobrachialis
7. subscapularis
8. serratus anterior
9. rhomboid minor
10. rhomboid major
11. supraspinatus
12. posterior deltoid
13. triceps (short head)
14. triceps (long head)
15. infraspinatus
16. teres minor
17. teres major

Movement: Scapula

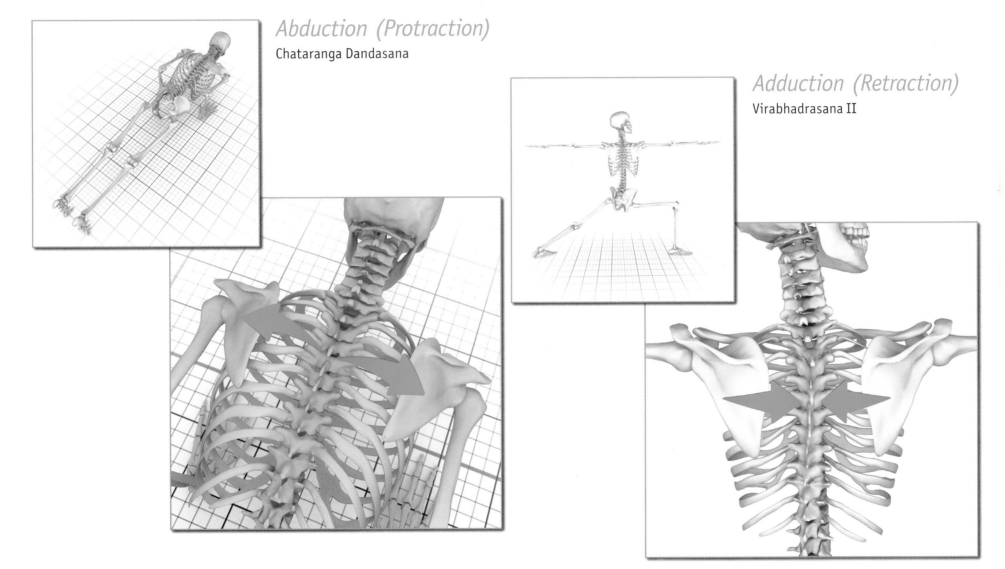

Abduction (Protraction)

Chataranga Dandasana

Adduction (Retraction)

Virabhadrasana II

Shoulder Girdle & Upper Arms

Movement: Scapula

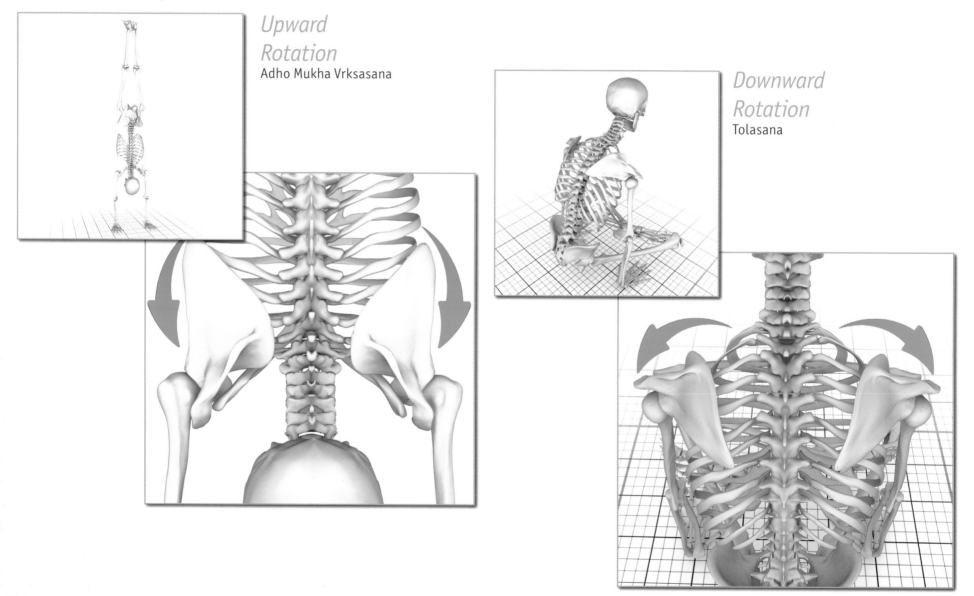

Upward Rotation
Adho Mukha Vrksasana

Downward Rotation
Tolasana

Movement: Upper Arm

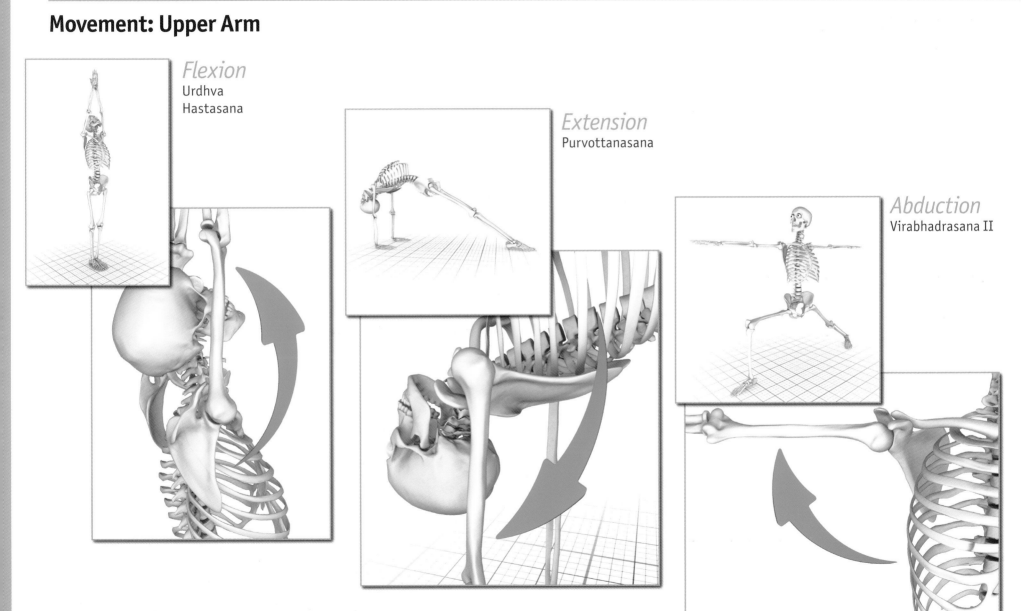

Flexion
Urdhva
Hastasana

Extension
Purvottanasana

Abduction
Virabhadrasana II

Movement: Upper Arm

Adduction
Vatayanasana

External Rotation
Gomukhasana B

Internal Rotation
Parsvottonasana

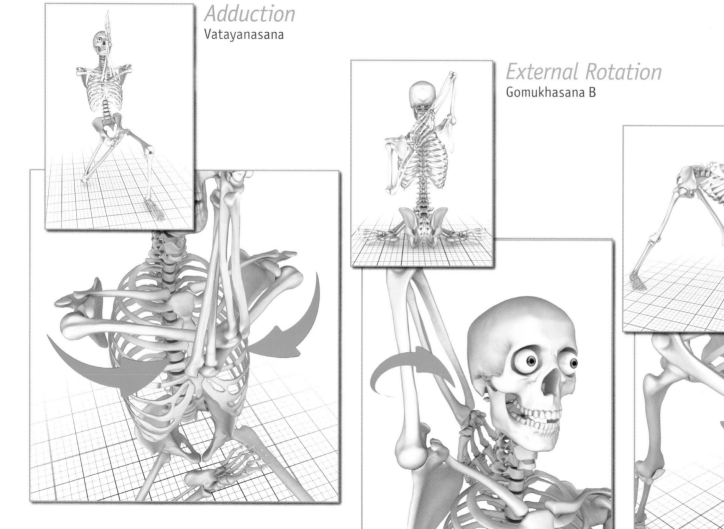

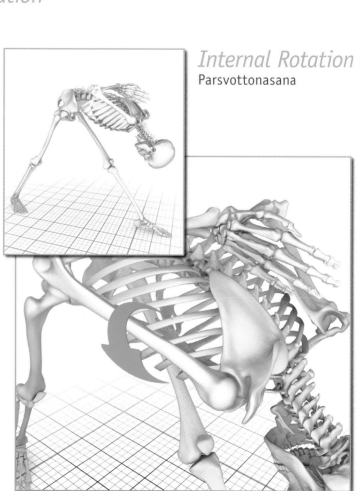

Chapter 14

Rhomboids

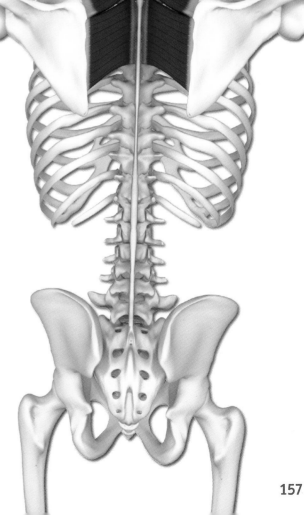

The major and minor rhomboids are flat rectangular muscles originating from the vertebral spinous processes and a ligament in the midline of the back and inserting on the medial border of the scapula. Contraction draws the scapula toward the midline and opens the chest. Postures such as Garudasana stretch the rhomboids. Contracting the rhomboids stabilizes the scapula and lifts the ribcage (in association with closed-chain contraction of the pectoralis minor). The rhomboids are direct antagonists of the serratus anterior muscle. The levator scapulae assist in lifting and rotating the scapulae.

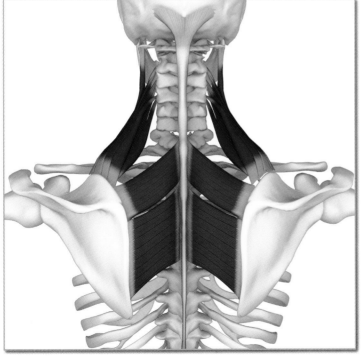

Rhomboids and Levator Scapulae

Rhomboids (rom-BOID)

Origin

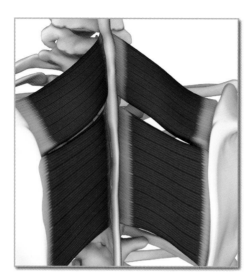

1) Major: Spinous processes of thoracic vertebrae 2 through 5 and the supraspinous ligament.

2) Minor: Spinous processes of cervical vertebra 7 and thoracic vertebra 1, lower ligamentum nuchae and supraspinous ligament.

Insertion

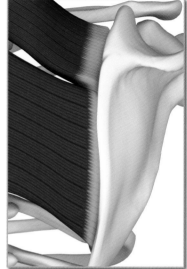

1) Major: Medial border from scapular spine to inferior angle of the scapula.

2) Minor: Upper medial border of the scapula.

Innervation & Chakra Illuminated

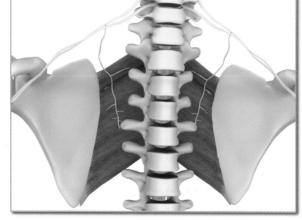

Dorsal scapular nerve (cervical nerve 5).

Chakra illuminated: Fifth.

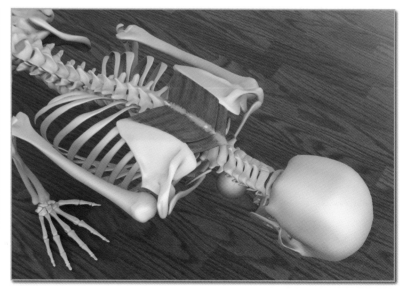

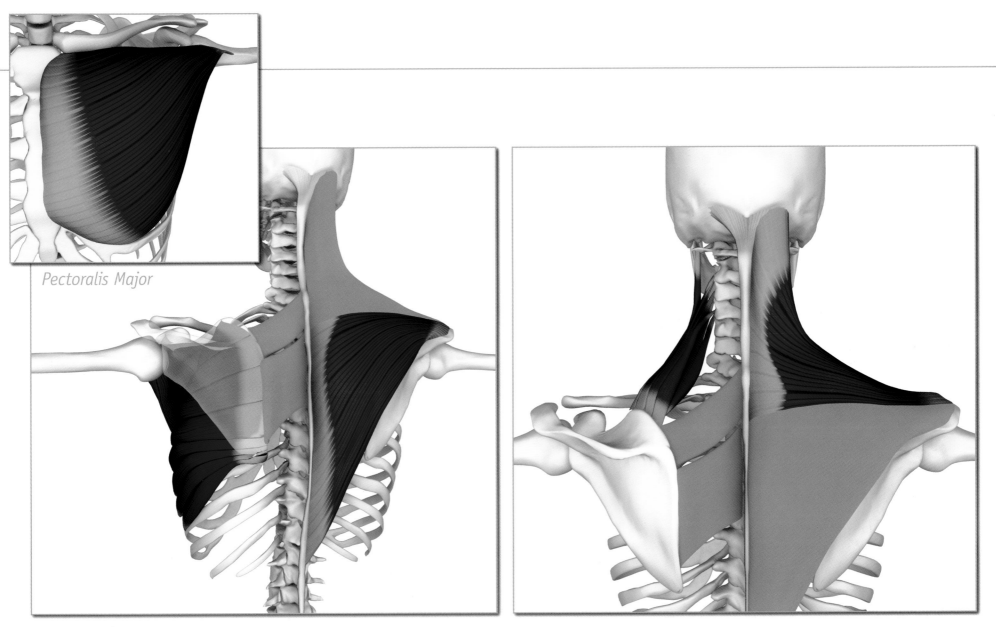

Pectoralis Major

Antagonists
Serratus anterior (seen here through the scapula), trapezius (lower fibers), and pectoralis major (sternocostal portion - see inset above).

Synergists
Levator scapulae and trapezius (upper fibers).

Rhomboids (rom-BOID)

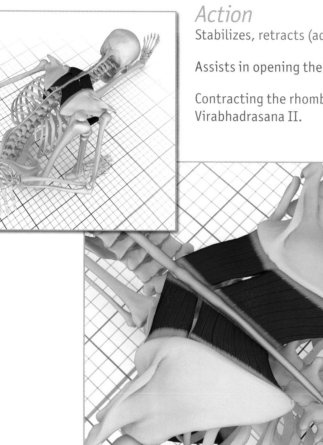

Action

Stabilizes, retracts (adducts), and rotates the scapulae downward.

Assists in opening the chest.

Contracting the rhomboids opens the chest in Marichyasana I and Virabhadrasana II.

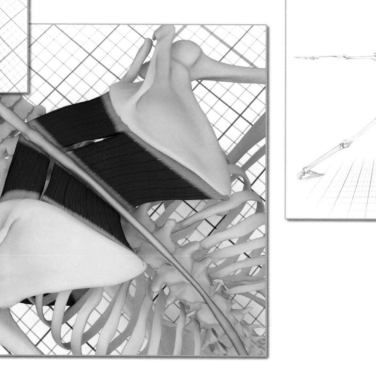

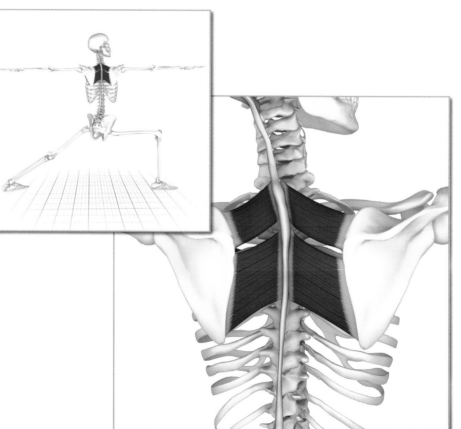

Contracted & Stretched

The rhomboids contract in Utthita Trikonasana, opposing the action of the serratus anterior (which also contracts). This action stabilizes the scapula and turns the chest.

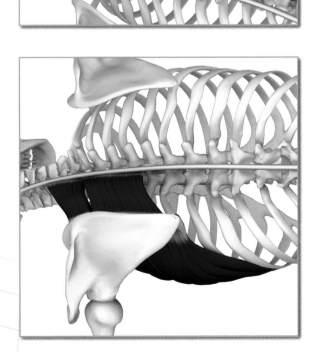

Chapter 15
Serratus Anterior

This multi-headed muscle forms the lateral part of the chest wall, giving it a "serrated" appearance. It originates from the superior borders of the upper nine ribs, inserting on the medial border of the scapula from the inside. Contracting this muscle draws the scapula forward and away from the midline, and relaxing it allows the scapula to be drawn toward the midline, opening the chest.

Weakness in the serratus anterior limits postures such as Chataranga Dandasana, resulting in the "winging" of the scapula (in which the medial borders lift off the back).

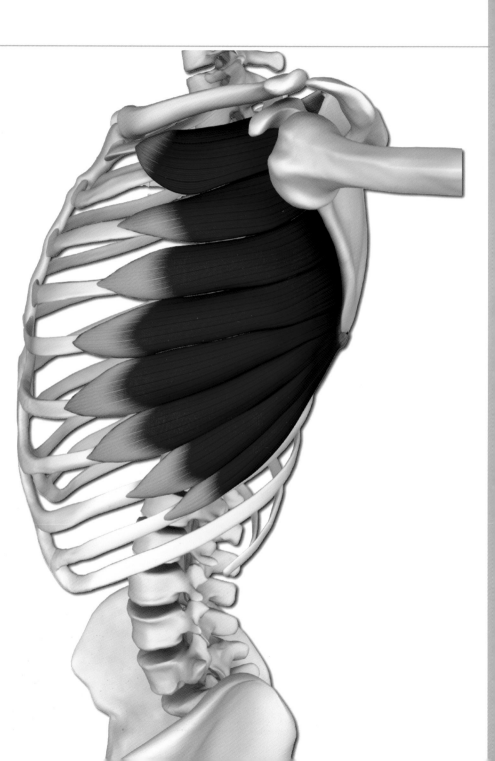

Serratus Anterior (ser-RA-tus an-TEER-I-or)

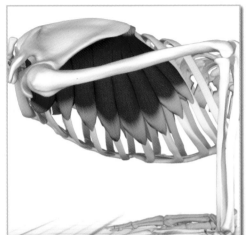

Origin

Outer surfaces and superior borders of ribs 1 through 9.

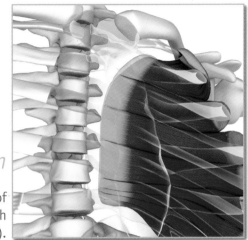

Insertion

Costal aspect of the medial border of the scapula (seen here through the chest).

Innervation & Chakra Illuminated

Long thoracic nerve (cervical nerves 5, 6, and 7).

Chakra illuminated: Fifth.

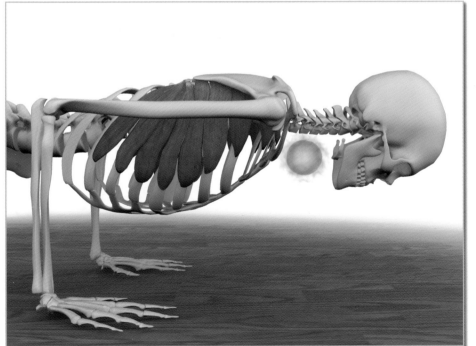

Serratus Anterior (ser-RA-tus an-TEER-I-or)

Antagonists

Rhomboid (major and minor) and trapezius (middle fibers).

Synergists

Pectoralis (major and minor).

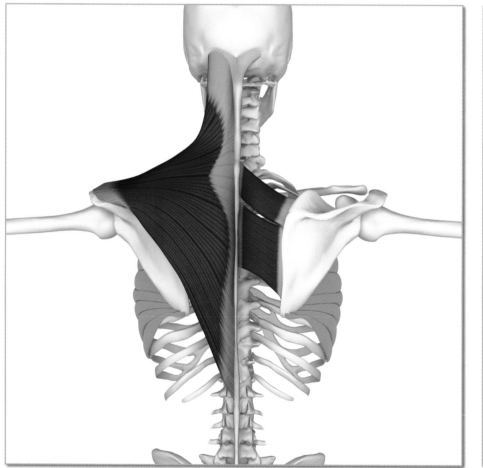

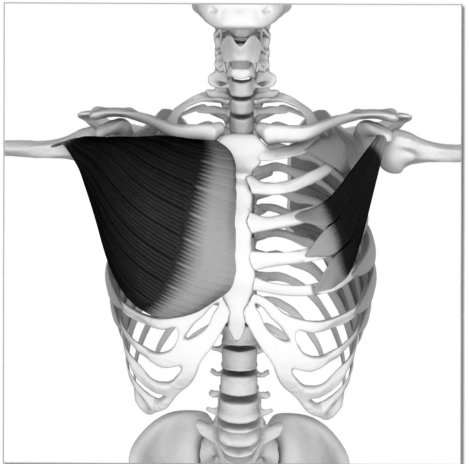

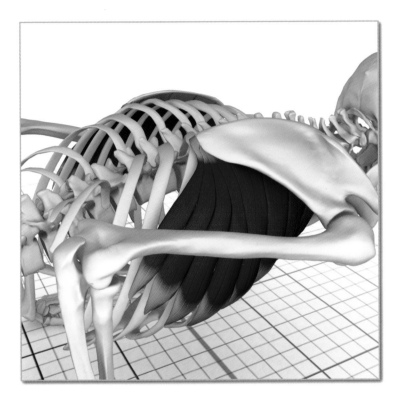

Action

Stabilizes and protracts (abducts) the scapulae, preventing the medial border from lifting or "winging" during pushing movements.

Assists scapular rotation.

The serratus anterior contracts and prevents "winging" of the scapulae in Chataranga Dandasana.

Serratus Anterior (ser-RA-tus an-TEER-I-or)

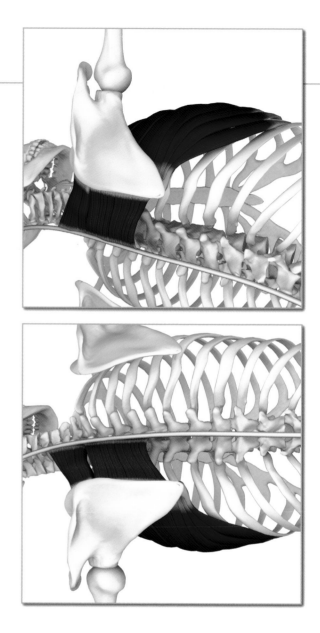

Contracted & Stretched

The serratus anterior muscles contract in Utthita Trikonasana, drawing the scapula away from the midline and extending the arms. This opposes the action of the rhomboids (which also contract in this pose). Adjusting the contraction of these opposing muscles assists in turning and opening the chest in this pose.

Chapter 16

Deltoids

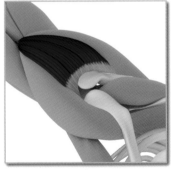

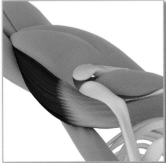

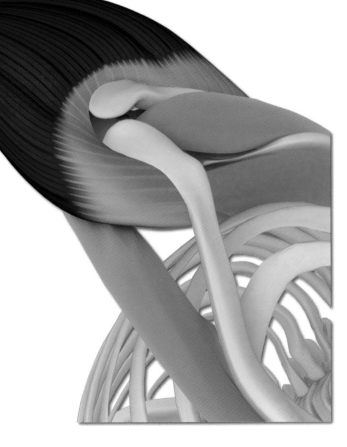

This is a three-part muscle with anterior, lateral, and posterior sections, originating from the clavicle, acromion, and scapulae, respectively, and inserting on the lateral humerus. The anterior section raises the arm forward. The posterior section extends the arm backward. These two sections are thus antagonists, and contracting one stretches the other. The lateral section abducts the arm.

Tightness in the anterior section limits postures in which the arm is extended backward, such as Purvottanasana. Tightness in the posterior section limits overhead movements such as Urdhva Danurasana and Virabhadrasana I. Tightness in the lateral section limits postures involving cross-body movements, such as Garudasana. Weakness in the deltoids limits postures in which the body weight is supported by the arms. Arm balances can be used to strengthen the deltoids.

Deltoids

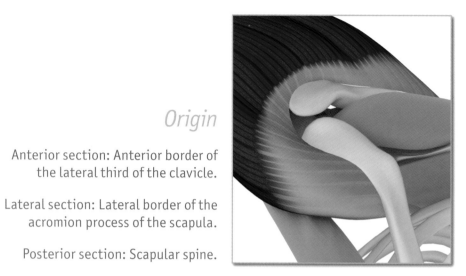

Origin

Anterior section: Anterior border of the lateral third of the clavicle.

Lateral section: Lateral border of the acromion process of the scapula.

Posterior section: Scapular spine.

Insertion

Deltoid tuberosity on the lateral surface of the humeral shaft.

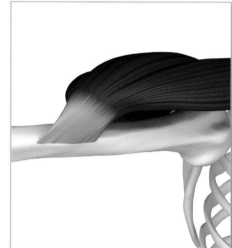

Innervation & Chakra Illuminated

Axillary nerve (cervical nerves 5 and 6).

Chakra illuminated: Fifth.

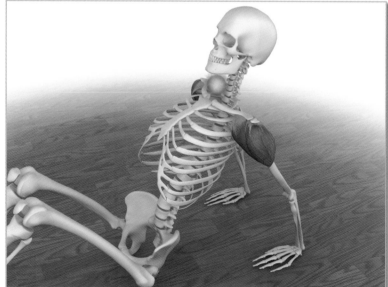

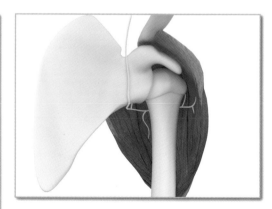

Deltoids–Anterior Section

Antagonists

Deltoids (posterior section), latissimus dorsi, and pectoralis major (sternocostal portion).

Synergists

Pectoralis major (clavicular portion).

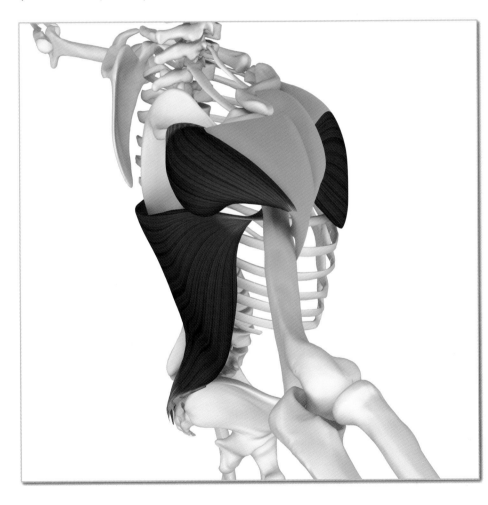

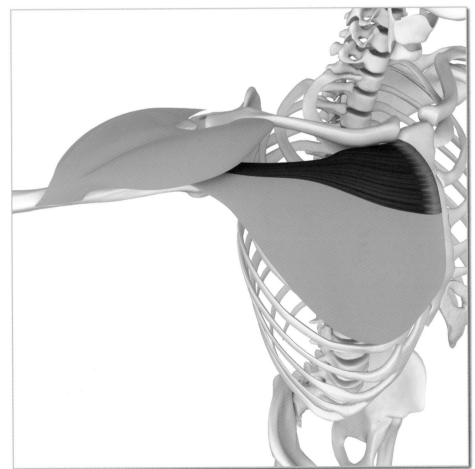

Deltoids–Lateral Section

Antagonists

Pectoralis major, latissimus dorsi, and triceps (long head).

Synergists

Supraspinatus and biceps (long head).

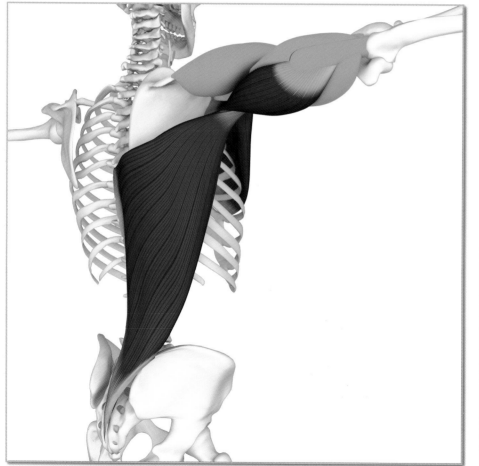

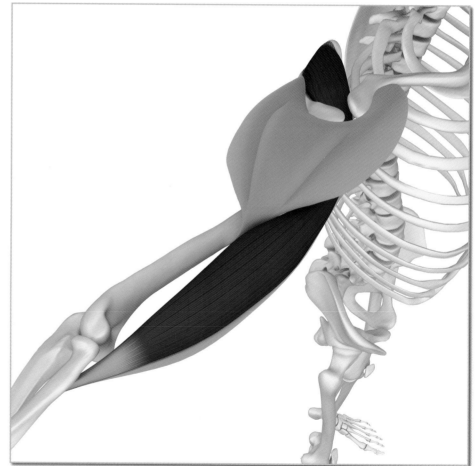

Deltoids–Posterior Section

Antagonists

Deltoids (anterior section), biceps (long head), and pectoralis major (clavicular portion).

Synergists

Latissimus dorsi and triceps (long head).

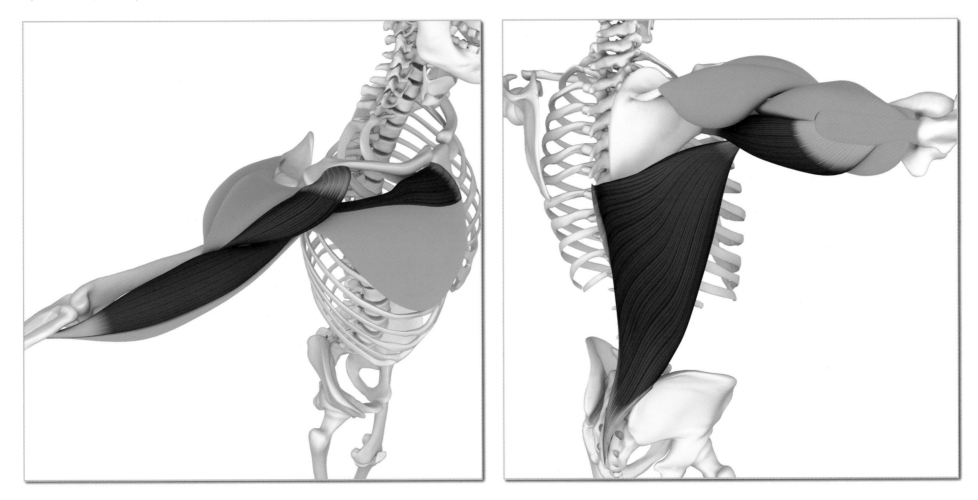

Deltoids (DEL-toid)

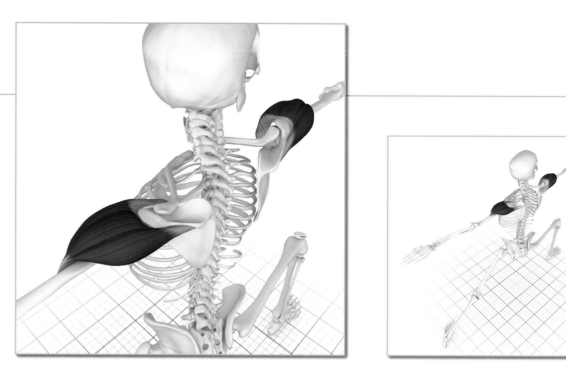

Action

The lateral section of the deltoids contracts in Virabhadrasana II, abducting the arms. The supraspinatus muscle of the rotator cuff initiates this action.

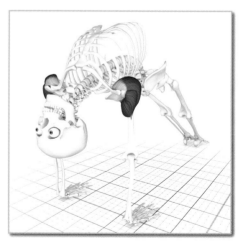

Awakening

The posterior section of the deltoids contracts, extending the arms in Purvottanasana and stretching the anterior deltoids, biceps brachii, and pectoralis major muscles.

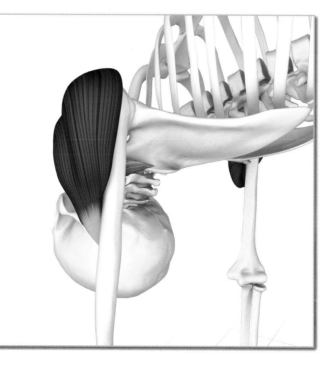

Contracted & Stretched

The lateral and posterior sections of the deltoids stretch in Vatayanasana. The pectoralis major contracts to accentuate this action.

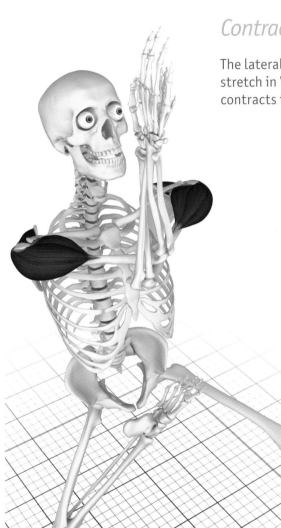

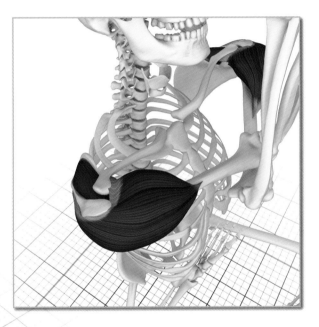

Contracted & Stretched

The anterior deltoid contracts in Adho Mukha Vrksasana, stretching the posterior deltoid, latissimus dorsi, and the lower fibers of the trapezius muscles.

Chapter 17

Rotator Cuff

The rotator cuff is a combination of four muscles: the subscapularis, the infraspinatus, the teres minor, and the supraspinatus. The subscapularis and infraspinatus have opposing actions and function as antagonists. The teres minor is a synergist of the infraspinatus and is not covered in detail here.

The shoulder (glenohumeral) joint is composed of a ball (the humeral head) and a shallow saucer-like socket (the glenoid of the scapula). The shoulder joint enjoys the greatest mobility of all the joints, but also has the least stability and is the joint most frequently dislocated. (Like a yin/yang, greater mobility means lesser stability.) The rotator cuff encircles the humeral head, stabilizing it within the shoulder joint.

As with the deep pelvic muscles, we are unaware of the rotator cuff, even though we use its muscles constantly in our daily life. Certain Yoga postures awaken our consciousness of these muscles. Once awakened, their contraction and relaxation can be used to refine other postures.

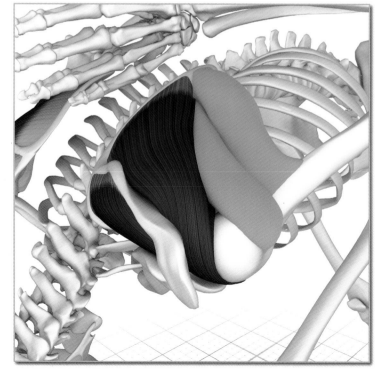

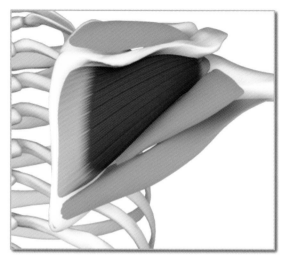

Infraspinatus (in-fruh-spi-NA-tus)

This muscle originates from the back (dorsal) surface of the scapula, inserting on the larger, more lateral greater tuberosity of the humerus. Contraction produces external rotation of the upper arm. The subscapularis and infraspinatus function as classic antagonists. Tightness of the infraspinatus limits internal rotation of the humerus, especially in postures such as Parsvottanasana. Weakness limits external rotation in poses such as Urdhva Danurasana.

Rotator Cuff

Supraspinatus (soo-pruh-spi-NA-tus)

The supraspinatus originates from the back (dorsal) surface of the scapula and inserts on the greater tuberosity of the humerus in front of the infraspinatus. The supraspinatus initiates arm abduction. Injury to this muscle results in the use of accessory muscles, such as the trapezius and deltoids, to accomplish this action.

Of all the rotator cuff muscles, the supraspinatus is the most frequently injured, due to impingement of its tendon on the inferior surface of the acromion process of the scapula. In Yoga, impingement can occur in Asanas such as dog pose and Urdhva Danurasana. This problem can be avoided by externally rotating the humerus and inwardly rotating the scapula.

Tightness of the supraspinatus limits poses where the arm crosses the chest (such as in Garudasana). Injuries may limit abduction of the arm, resulting in a "shrugged" shoulder appearance to poses where the arm is abducted (such as Virabhadrasana II).

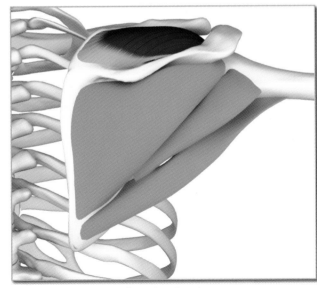

Supraspinatus (back view)

Subscapularis (sub-skap-u-LARE-us)

The subscapularis originates from the inside (ventral) surface of the scapula and inserts on a knob-shaped structure called the "lesser tuberosity" of the humeral head. Contracting the subscapularis internally rotates the humerus. Tightness in this muscle limits poses with an external rotation component of the upper arms, such as Urdhva Danurasana. Weakness limits poses such as Parsvottanasana.

Rotator Cuff

Origin
Subscapularis

Subscapular fossa on the anterior surface of the scapula (seen here through the chest).

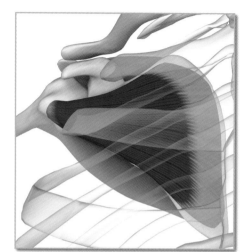

Insertion
Subscapularis

Lesser tuberosity of the humerus and capsule of the shoulder joint (lower part).

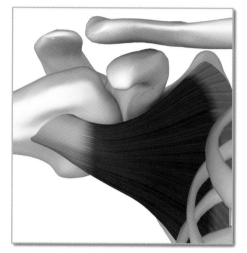

Origin
Infraspinatus

Infraspinous fossa of the scapula.

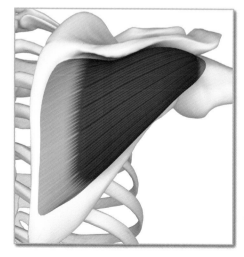

Insertion
Infraspinatus

Middle facet of the greater tuberosity of the humerus and capsule of the shoulder joint (shown from above).

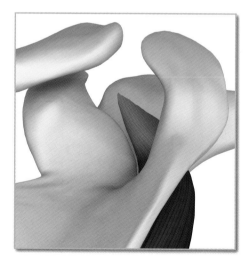

Origin
Supraspinatus
(back view)

Supraspinous fossa of the scapula.

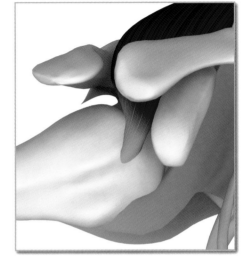

Insertion
Supraspinatus
(front view)

Upper part of the greater tuberosity of the humerus and capsule of the shoulder joint.

Innervation & Chakra Illuminated

Subscapularis: Upper and lower subscapular nerves (cervical nerves 5 and 6).

Infraspinatus: Suprascapular nerve (cervical nerves 5 and 6).

Supraspinatus: Suprascapular nerve (cervical nerves 5 and 6).

Chakra illuminated: Fifth.

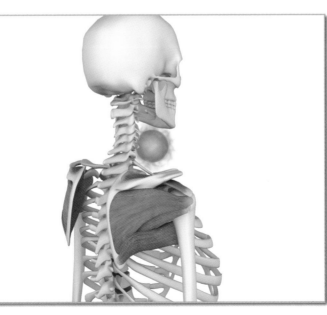

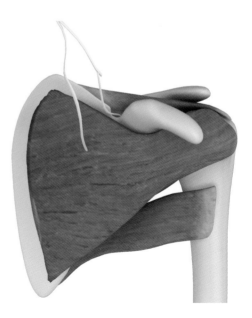

Subscapularis

Antagonists

Infraspinatus, posterior deltoid, and teres minor.

Synergists

Pectoralis major, latissimus dorsi, and anterior deltoid.

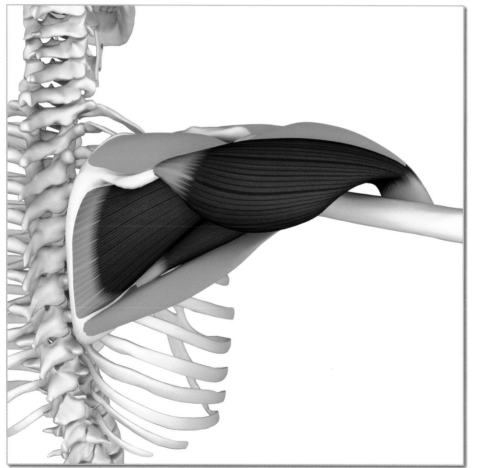

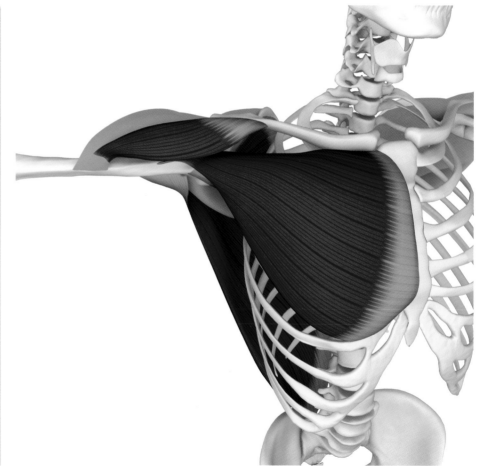

Infraspinatus

Antagonists

Subscapularis, latissimus dorsi, pectoralis major, and anterior deltoid.

Synergists

Teres minor and posterior deltoid.

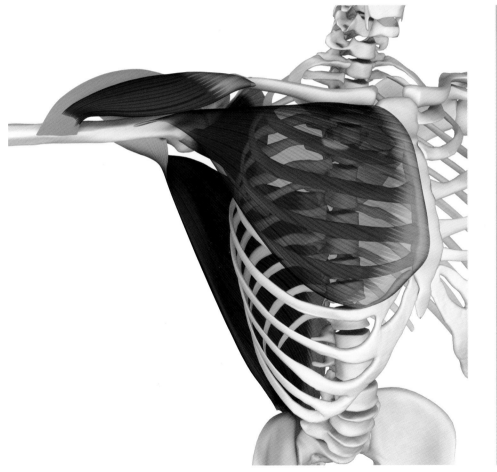
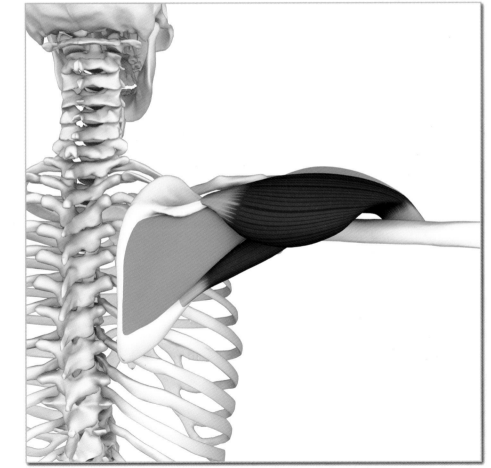

Supraspinatus

Antagonists

Pectoralis major, latissimus dorsi, and triceps (long head).

Synergists

Lateral deltoid and biceps (long head).

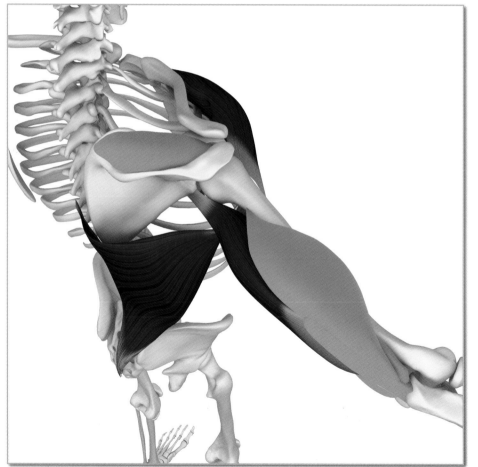

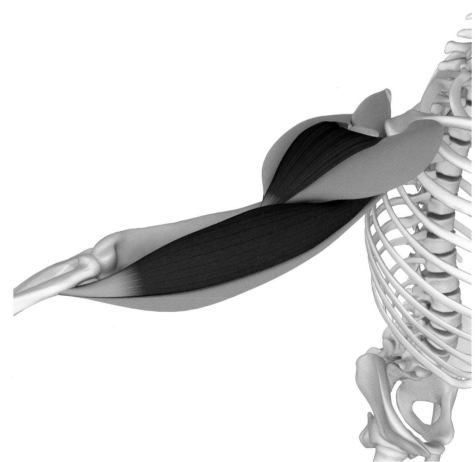

Subscapularis & Infraspinatus

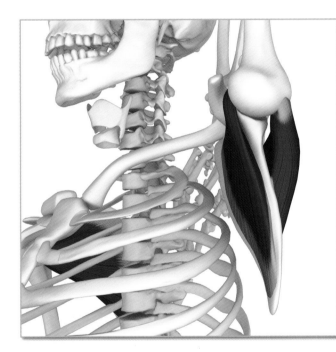

Contracted & Stretched

Gomukhasana B: The upper arm infraspinatus contracts, stretching the subscapularis. The lower arm subscapularis contracts, stretching the infraspinatus.

Supraspinatus

Contracted

The supraspinatus abducts the arm and stabilizes the glenohumeral joint.

Contraction of the supraspinatus initiates abduction in Virabhadrasana II. The lateral section of the deltoid accentuates and sustains this action.

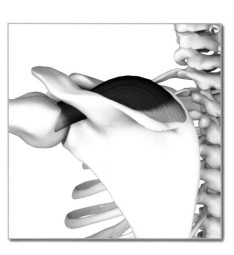

Stretched

The supraspinatus stretches in Vatayanasana. Drawing the upper arm further across the body toward the opposite side (by contracting the same-side pectoralis major) accentuates this action.

Shoulder Biomechanics

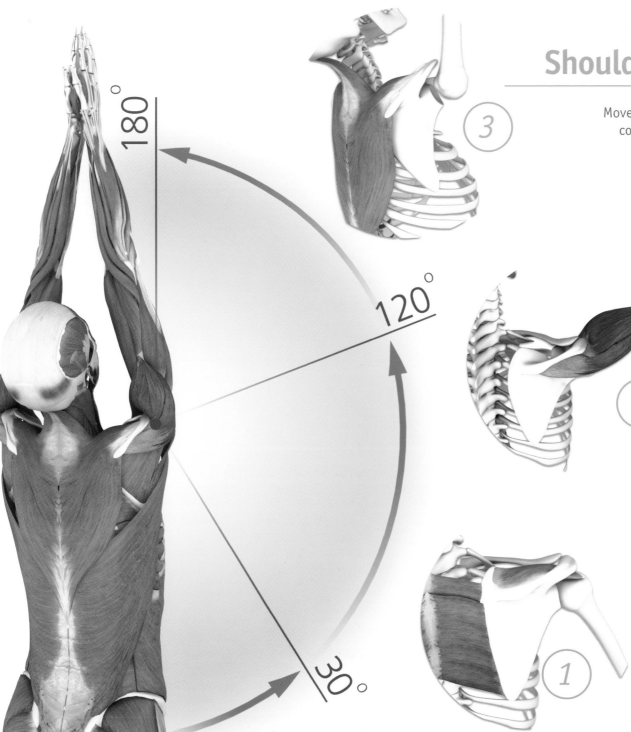

Movement of the shoulder takes place through coupling of three separate joints: the glenohumeral, scapulothoracic, and acromioclavicular joints.

Shoulder abduction and elevation of the humerus begins by stabilizing the scapula.

1. The supraspinatus initiates abduction at the glenohumeral joint.

2. The deltoid sustains glenohumeral abduction to approximately 120°.

3. The trapezius completes abduction of the shoulder by outwardly rotating the scapula.

This movement is apparent in the various Yoga postures where the arm is elevated or abducted.

Impingement

The subacromial bursa is a sac-like, fluid-filled structure that facilitates the gliding of the rotator cuff under the acromion. Impingement involves compression of the subacromial bursa between the greater tuberosity of the humerus and the acromion. This can result in shoulder pain.

Contracting the infraspinatus externally rotates the humerus and draws the greater tuberosity away from the acromion. Contracting the long head of the triceps rotates the acromion toward the midline, away from the greater tuberosity. Contracting both of these muscles creates space between the acromion and the greater tuberosity, assisting to prevent impingement of the bursa.

Contract these muscles to externally rotate the humerus and outwardly rotate the scapula when performing postures involving overhead movements.

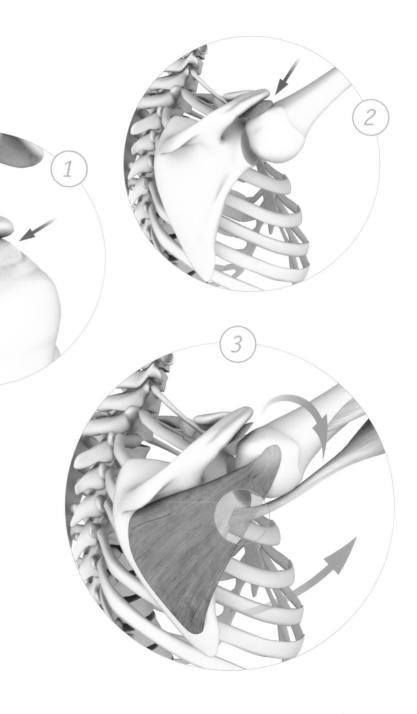

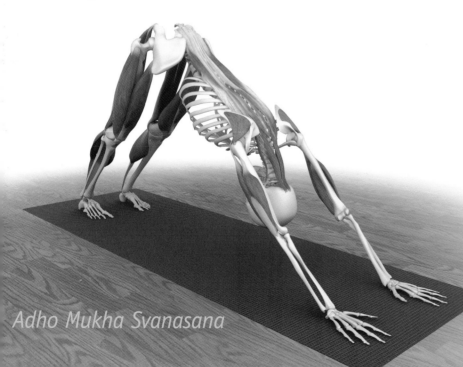

Adho Mukha Svanasana

Chapter 18
Biceps Brachii

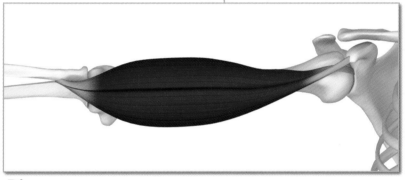

Biceps

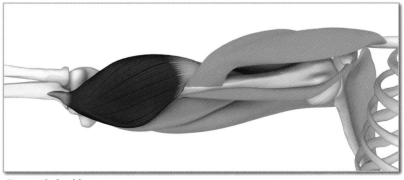

Brachialis

This is a two-headed fusiform muscle. The short head originates from the coracoid (crow's beak) process of the scapula, near the insertion of the pectoralis minor. When the elbow is fixed, contracting the short head tilts the scapula forward. The long head originates from the top of the glenoid of the scapula, curving over the humeral head and into the bicipital groove (a trough into which it is tethered by a ligament). Contracting the long head with the elbow fixed depresses the humeral head, stabilizing it in the joint.

Both heads combine to form one tendon that inserts on the bicipital tuberosity of the radius. When the biceps contract, the forearm rotates into supination (palm up). Further contraction flexes the elbow.

Tightness in this muscle limits poses such as Purvottanasana. Weakness limits poses such as Sarvangasana.

The brachialis muscle acts in synergy with the biceps, flexing the elbow.

Biceps Brachii (BI-seps BRA-ke-I)

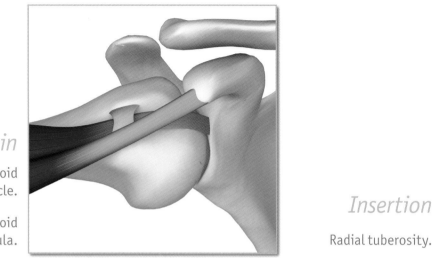

Origin

Long Head: Supraglenoid
tubercle.

Short Head: Tip of the coracoid
process of the scapula.

Insertion

Radial tuberosity.

Innervation & Chakra Illuminated

Musculocutaneous nerve (cervical nerves 5 and 6).
Chakra illuminated: Fifth.

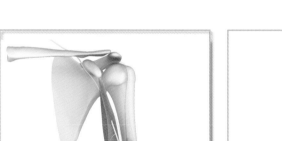

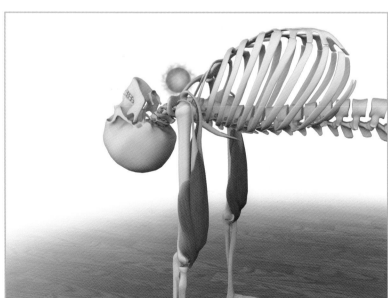

Antagonists

Triceps and posterior deltoid.

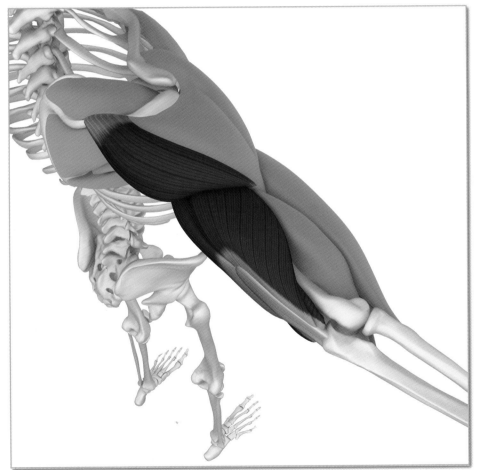

Synergists

Anterior deltoid and pectoralis major (sternocostal portion).

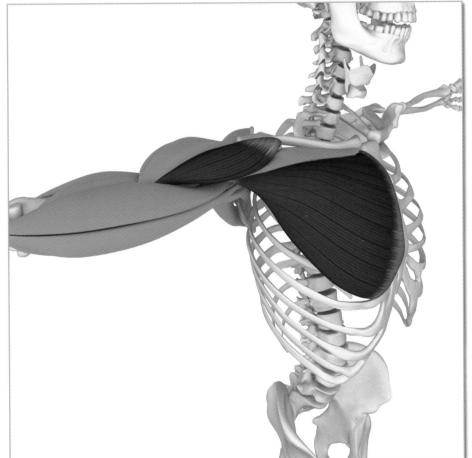

Biceps Brachii (BI-seps BRA-ke-I)

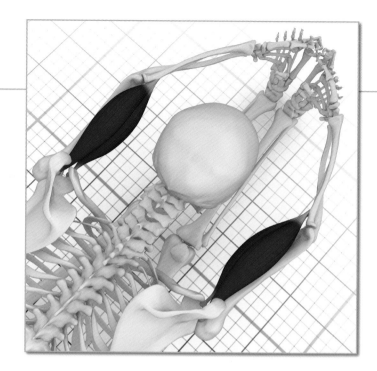

Contracted

The biceps contract, flexing the elbows to draw the upper body forward in Paschimottanasana. The force produced by this action ultimately affects the position of the pelvis, tilting it forward. This draws the ischial tuberosities backward, stretching the hamstrings.

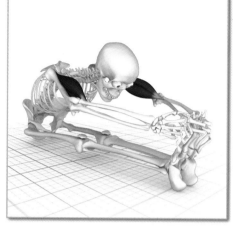

Stretched

The biceps stretch in Purvottanasana. The triceps and posterior section of the deltoids contract to accentuate this action.

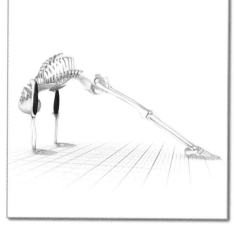

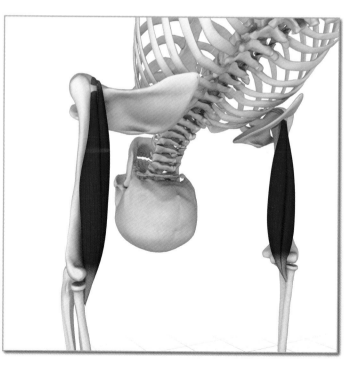

Action & Awakening

The biceps contract, flexing the elbow and supinating the forearm in Sarvangasana. This action stabilizes the back, strengthening the biceps and brachialis.

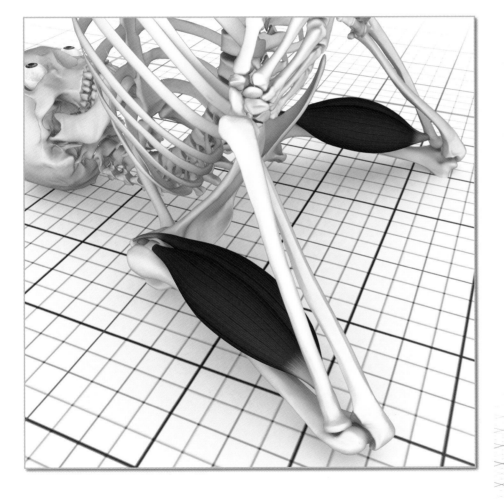

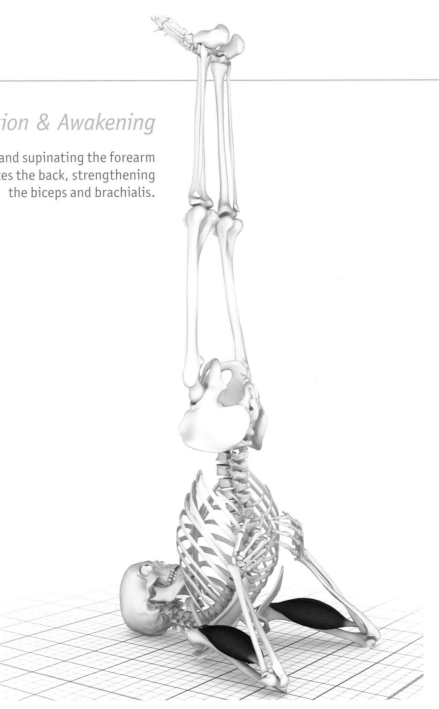

Chapter 19
Triceps Brachii

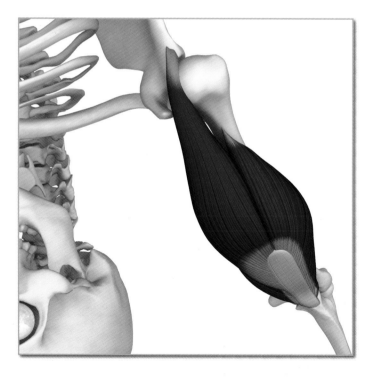

The triceps brachii is a three-headed muscle on the back of the arm. The medial and short heads originate from the humerus. The long head originates from the inferior border of the glenoid. All three heads combine to form one distal tendon that inserts on the olecranon process of the ulna (forearm bone).

Contraction of all three heads extends the elbow (as in Downward Facing Dog pose). Contraction of the long head with the forearm fixed rotates the scapula upward (by pulling on its origin). This rotation increases contact of the humeral head with the shallow glenoid, stabilizing the joint. This contraction of the triceps also moves the acromion process medially and away from the humeral head, preventing impingement of the acromion on the humeral head. This protects the rotator cuff muscles in poses like back bends and Downward Dog.

Contraction of the triceps opens the front of the elbow (antebrachial fossa) and relieves blockages in the minor Chakra of the elbow. Weakness in the triceps limits the ability to perform various arm balances.

Triceps Brachii (TRI-seps BRA-ke-I)

Origin

1) *Lateral Head:* Upper half of the posterior surface of the humeral shaft.

2) *Medial Head:* Posterior shaft of the humerus, distal to the radial groove.

3) *Long Head:* Infraglenoid tubercle of the scapula (looking into the armpit).

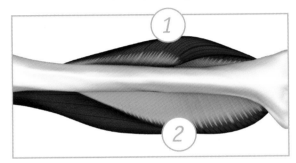

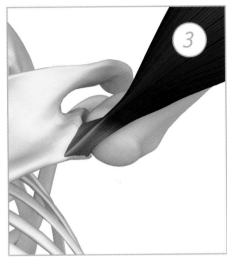

Insertion

Posterior surface of the olecranon process of the ulna (back view).

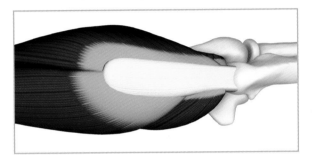

Innervation & Chakra Illuminated

Radial nerve (cervical nerves 7 and 8).

Chakra illuminated: Fifth.

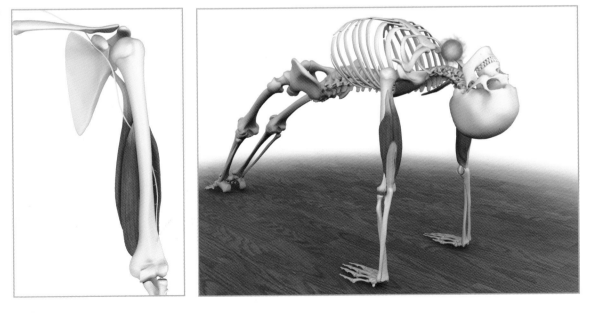

Triceps Brachii (TRI-seps BRA-ke-I)

Antagonists

Biceps and anterior deltoid.

Synergists

Latissimus dorsi and posterior deltoid.

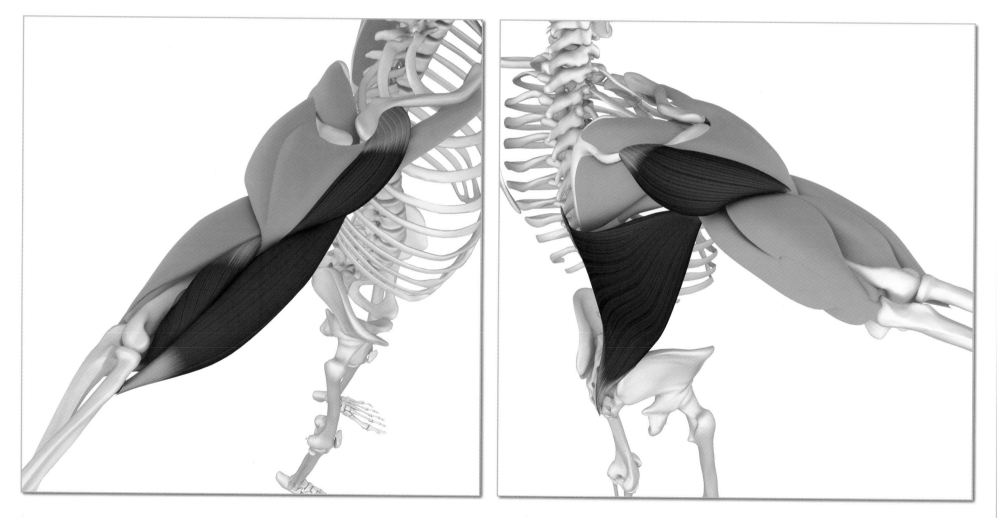

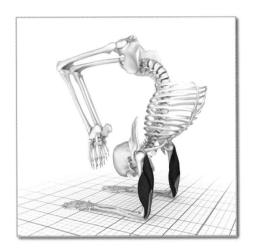

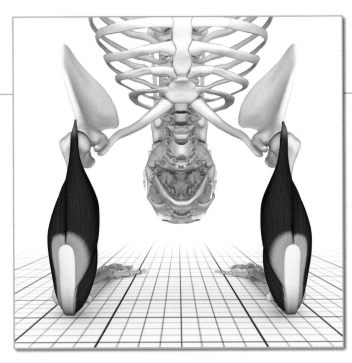

Contracted

The triceps contract and stabilize the upper arms and shoulders in Vrishchikasana (and similar Asanas such as Pincha Mayurasana).

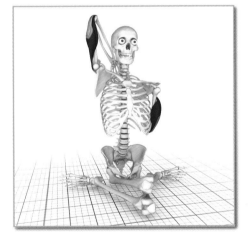

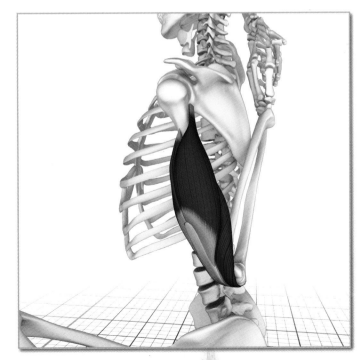

Stretched

The upper and lower arm triceps stretch in Gomukhasana B.

Triceps Brachii (TRI-seps BRA-ke-I)

Action & Awakening

The triceps contract, extending the elbows in Urdhva Danurasana.

The long head of the triceps also upwardly rotates the scapula, increasing contact between the humeral head and the glenoid. This aids to prevent impingement of the humeral head on the acromion.

The triceps contract, extending the elbows in Urdhva Mukha Svanasana. The force produced by this action assists in extending the knees and stretching the hamstrings.

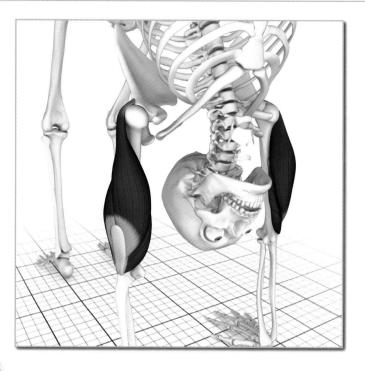

Test your anatomy*

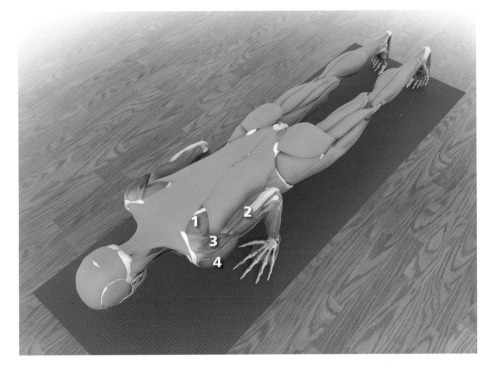

1. biceps brachi
2. triceps long head
3. triceps
4. serratus anterior
5. posterior deltoid
6. levator scapula

1. rhomboid
2. biceps brachii
3. infra spinatus
4. posterior deltoid

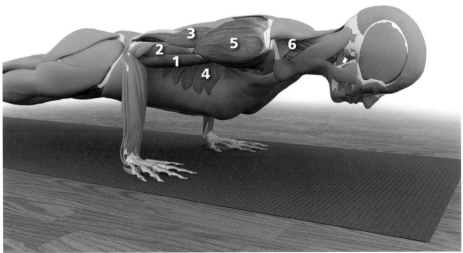

Test your anatomy*

1 triceps
2 biceps
3 Serratus anterias
4 trapezius
5 Postrica deltoid
6 anterior deltoid

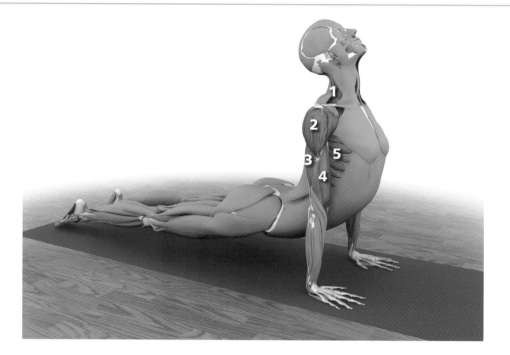

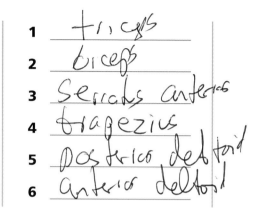

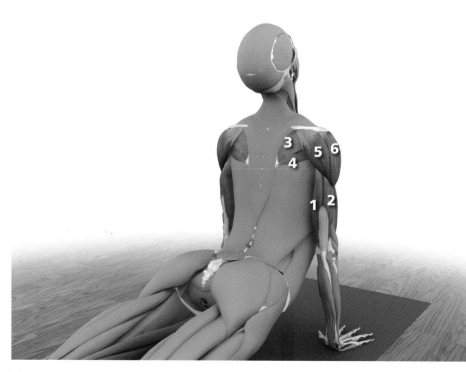

1 levator scapulae
2 lateral deltoid
3 triceps
4 biceps
5 Serratus anterias

*Please see www.BandhaYoga.com for answers...

Chapter20
Sternocleidomastoid

This is a two-headed strap-like muscle located on both sides of the front of the neck. It originates from the sternum and clavicle, inserting on the skull, behind the ear (the mastoid process).

Contracting the sternocleidomastoid when the head is fixed lifts the ribcage. It flexes the neck forward when the head is mobile. Contracting one side tilts the head to the same side and turns the head to the opposite side, stretching the contralateral muscle.

This muscle is important in creating the lock formed in Jalandhara Bandha and assists in lifting the ribcage during respiration. Tightness limits turning or extending the head as in Utthita Trikonasana or Purvottanasana, respectively.

Sternocleidomastoid (ster-no-kli-do-MAS-toid)

Origin

Manubrium of sternum and medial section of the clavicle.

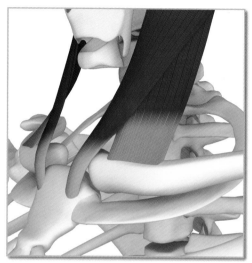

Insertion

Mastoid process.

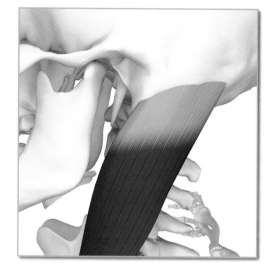

Innervation & Chakra Illuminated

Spinal accessory nerve (cranial nerve 11 and cervical nerves 2 and 3).

Chakra illuminated: Fifth.

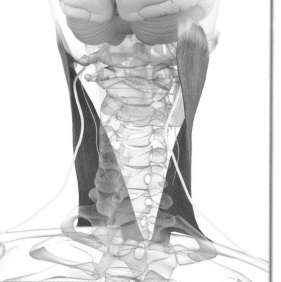

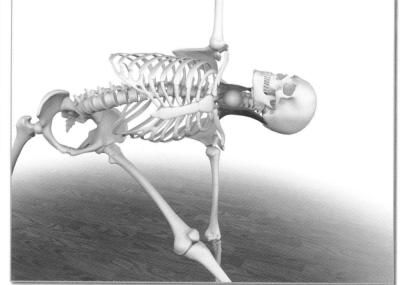

Antagonists

Trapezius and dorsal neck muscles.

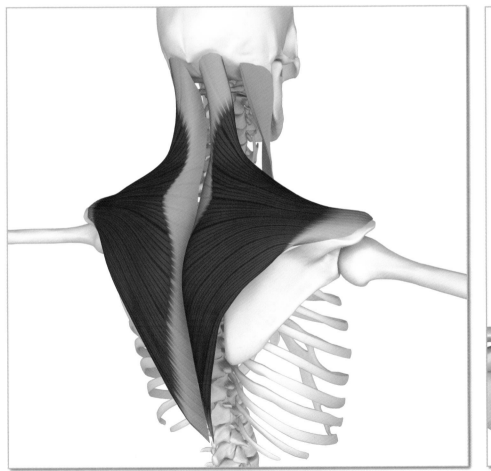

Synergists

Sterno thyreoideus and scaleni.

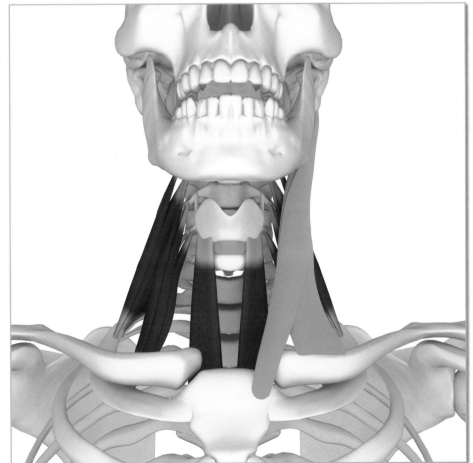

Sternocleidomastoid (ster-no-kli-do-MAS-toid)

Action & Awakening

Bilateral contraction:
Flexes the neck forward and draws the chin downward.

Unilateral contraction:
Rotates and tilts the head to face the opposite side.

Closed-chain contraction lifts the ribcage during respiration.

The sternocleidomastoid contracts, drawing the head forward to the sternum in Padmasana. This action lifts the ribcage, accentuating Jalandhara Bandha.

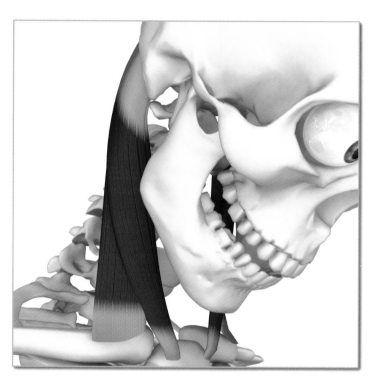

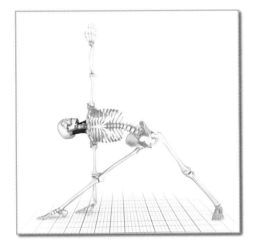

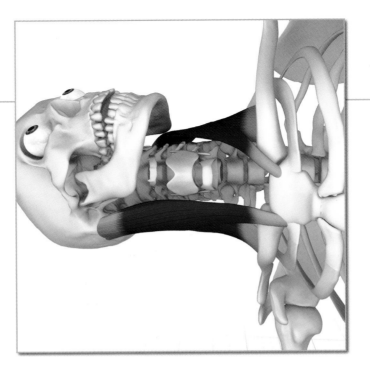

Contracted

The lower-side sternocleidomastoid contracts in Utthita Trikonasana, lengthening the upper-side sternocleidomastoid and turning the head.

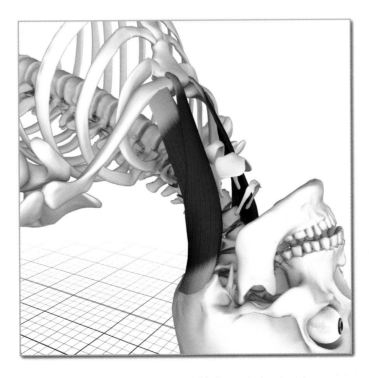

Stretched

The dorsal neck muscles and upper trapezius contract in Purvottanasana, stretching both sternocleidomastoid muscles.

Chapter 21

Lower Leg and Foot

The lower leg and foot form the foundation for many Yoga poses. For this reason, it is important to have a functional understanding of the major muscles of the lower leg and foot. Minor Chakras in the foot contribute to illuminating the first and second major Chakras.

For ease of understanding, it is useful to divide the many muscles in this region into groups identified by their function.

The major functions include flexing, extending, everting, and inverting the foot. In the foot itself, the muscles are categorized into flexors and extensors of the toes.

These illustrations demonstrate the major muscles performing these actions.

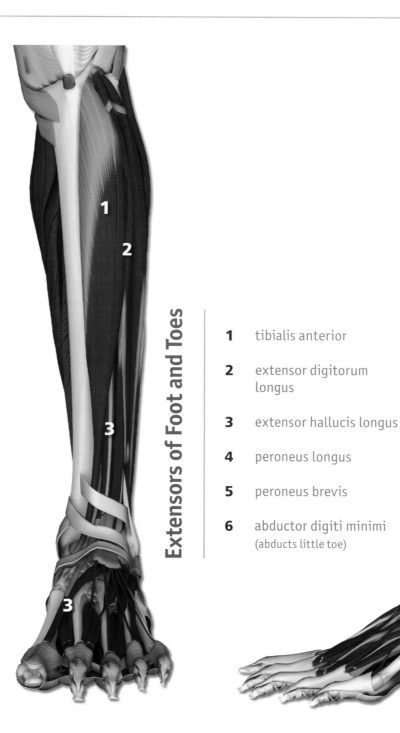

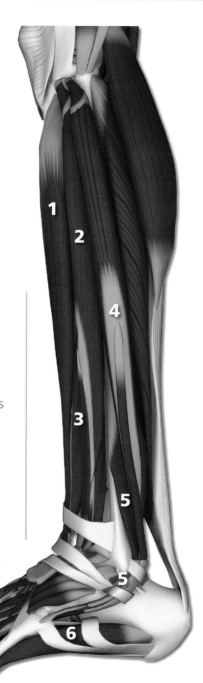

Extensors of Foot and Toes

1   tibialis anterior

2   extensor digitorum longus

3   extensor hallucis longus

4   peroneus longus

5   peroneus brevis

6   abductor digiti minimi
    (abducts little toe)

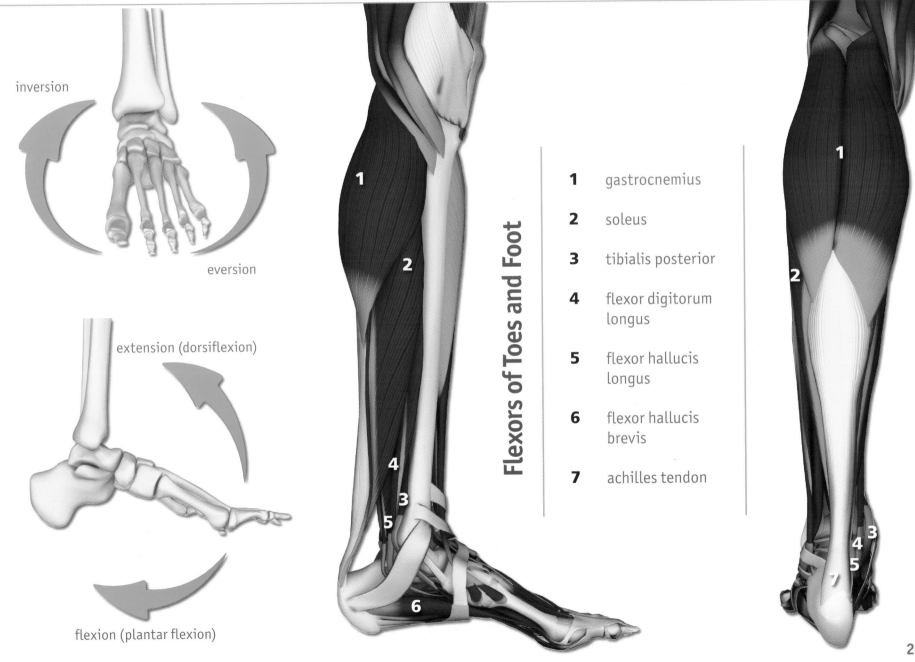

inversion

eversion

extension (dorsiflexion)

flexion (plantar flexion)

Flexors of Toes and Foot

1 gastrocnemius

2 soleus

3 tibialis posterior

4 flexor digitorum longus

5 flexor hallucis longus

6 flexor hallucis brevis

7 achilles tendon

Movement: Foot

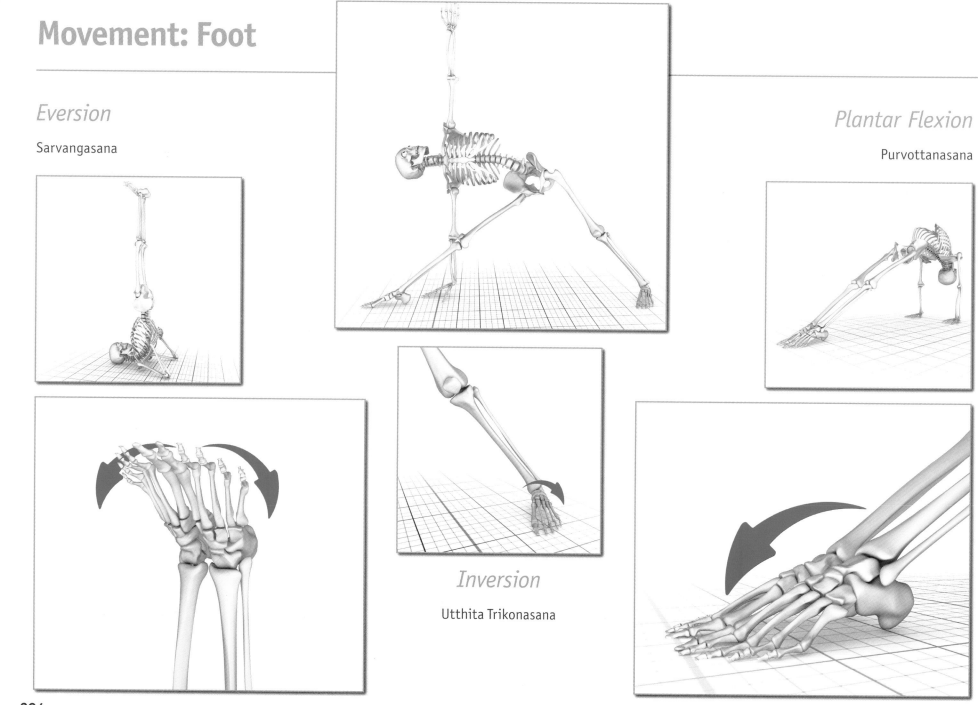

Eversion

Sarvangasana

Plantar Flexion

Purvottanasana

Inversion

Utthita Trikonasana

Gastrocnemius

The gastrocnemius is a two-headed fusiform muscle originating from the backs of the femoral condyles and inserting on the calcaneus (heel bone) via the Achilles tendon. Its primary action is plantar flexion of the foot. The gastrocnemius also acts synergistically with the hamstrings to flex the knee during the push-off phase of walking, propelling the body forward.

Tightness in the gastrocnemius limits extension of the knee (as with tightness in the hamstrings). Facilitated stretching of the gastrocnemius is an effective method to break through limitations in forward-bending postures where the knees straighten.

Use the forward bend Paschimottanasana to bring the gastrocnemius out to full length, and then resist plantar flexion of the feet by pulling them toward the head with the hands. Hold this for a few moments, and then extend the knees and draw the feet upward.

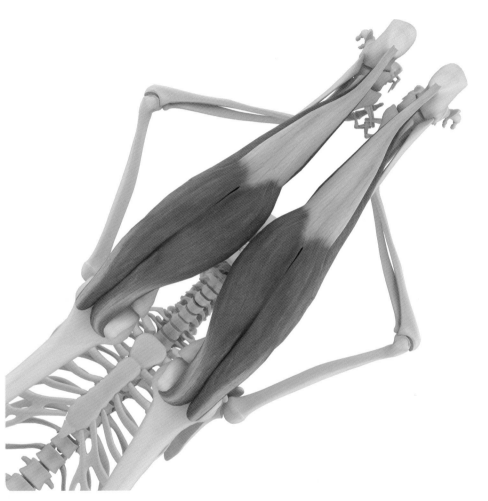

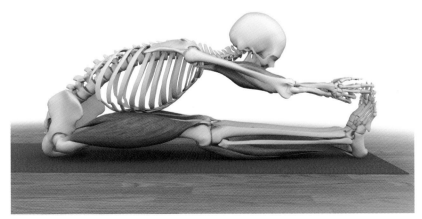

Paschimottanasana

This view from the floor illustrates the polyarticular nature of the gastrocnemius and how it originates from the posterior femoral condyles, crosses the knee, and inserts on the calcaneus (via the achilles tendon).

Paschimottanasana illustrates stretching the gastrocnemius by contracting the quadriceps to extend the knees. The hands dorsiflex the ankles.

Chapter 22

Forearm & Hand

The muscles of the forearm and hand connect the upper body with the lower body in Yoga. They also stabilize the body in balancing poses and inversions. Minor Chakras are present in the hand that illumniate the fourth and fifth major Chakras.

For ease of understanding, it is useful to divide the many muscles in this region into groups identified by their function.

The major functions include flexing and extending the wrist and complex movements of the hand and fingers. This chapter illustrates the flexors and extensors of this region.

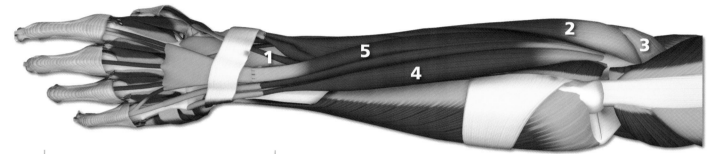

Extensors

1	extensor pollicis longus
2	extensor carpi radialis brevis
3	extensor carpi radialis longus
4	extensor carpi ulnaris
5	extensor digitorum

Flexors

6	flexor carpi ulnaris
7	flexor digitorum profundus (deep to palmaris longus)
8	brachioradialis
9	flexor digitorum superficialis
10	flexor carpi radialis

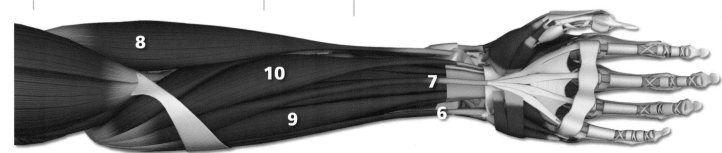

Movement

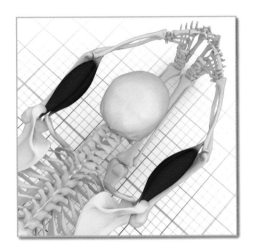

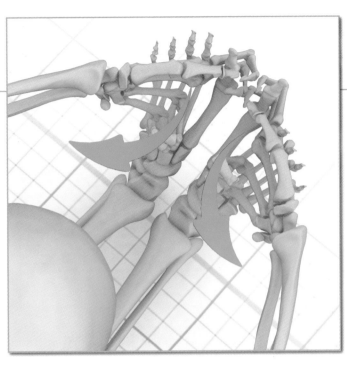

Flexed

The fingers, wrists, and forearms flex to grip the feet and draw the body deeper into forward bends.

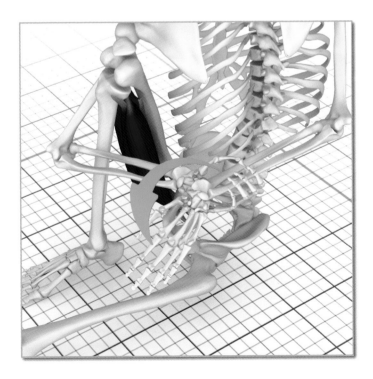

Extended

Extending the wrist can be used to form a lock behind the back in twisting poses.

Forearm & Hand

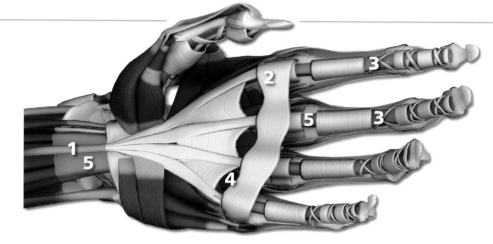

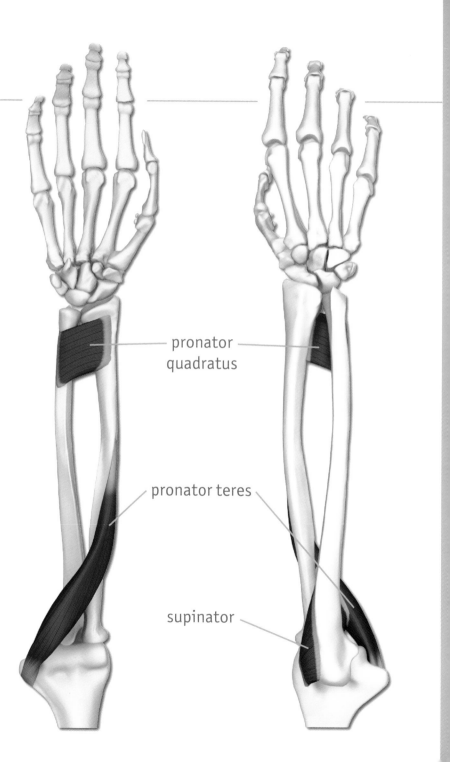

1. **1**   palmaris longus
2. **2**   palmar arch
3. **3**   flexor digitorum profundus
4. **4**   intrinsic muscles (adductors and abductors)

5. **5**   flexor digitorum superficialis
6. **6**   extensor and abductor pollicis
7. **7**   extensor digitorum
8. **8**   extensor digiti minimi
9. **9**   digital sheaths

pronator quadratus

pronator teres

supinator

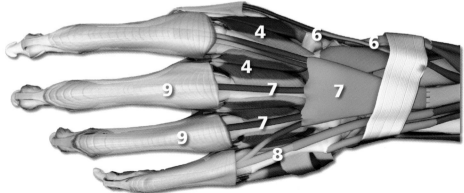

Movement

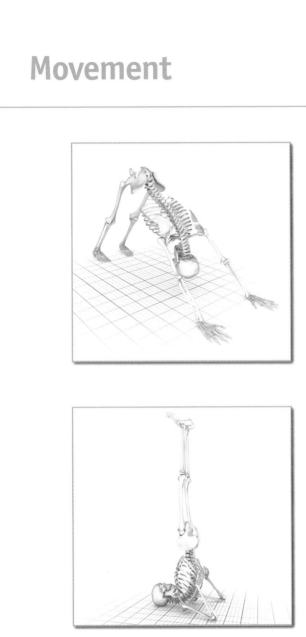

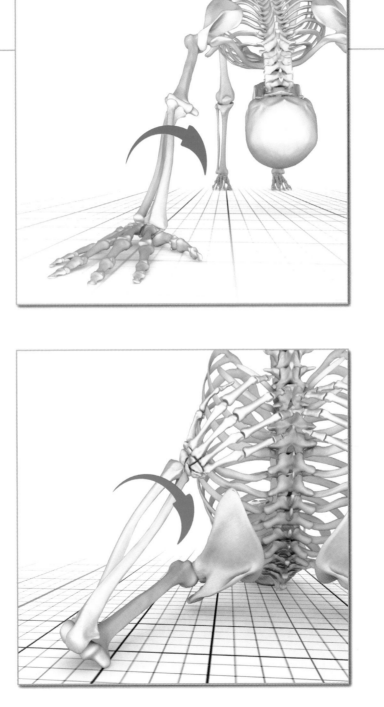

Pronation

The pronator teres and pronator quadratus muscles of the forearm contract, turning the palm down.

Supination

The biceps brachii and supinator muscles contract, turning the palm up.

Chapter 23
Myofascial & Organ Planes

A connective tissue sheath encapsulates and separates individual muscles and organs. A thin layer of body fluid coats these sheaths, facilitating the gliding of muscles over neighboring structures. This fluid is apparent in the shiny appearance of muscles and organs during surgery.

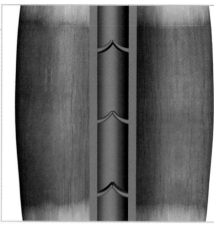

The One-Way Valve System

Massage stimulates nerves and mobilizes fluids within the myofascial and organ planes. Contraction and relaxation of muscles during Yoga practice has a similar effect on nerve conduction and fluid transport. The pumping action of the muscles propels body fluids through the one-way valve system of the vessels.

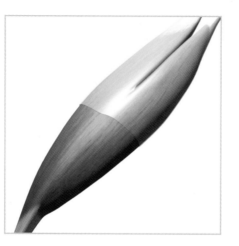

The Myofascial Planes

The space between the muscles is called the myofascial plane. Blood vessels, nerves, and lymphatics lie in this space and within the connective tissue sheaths themselves.

Blood vessels and lymphatics have one-way valves that direct the flow of body fluids to the larger central vessels. Toxins within the blood and lymphatic fluid are then transported to lymph nodes and organs, such as the liver, facilitating their removal.

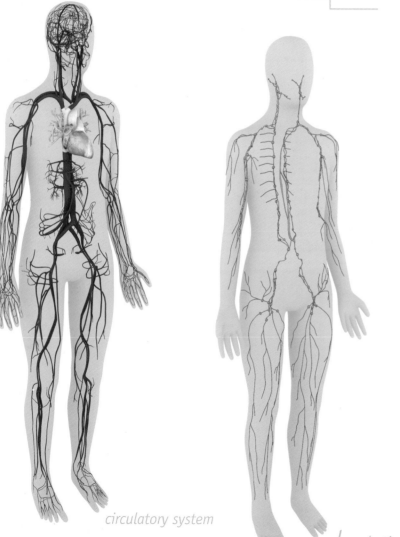

circulatory system

lymphatic system

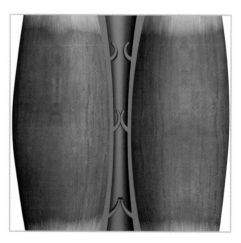

Fascia

The fascial planes are a lattice-like matrix of thin sheets of connective tissue that cover the organs and muscles. Sensory nerves are found throughout the various fascial planes and are stimulated by stretching the fascia in Yoga postures. This nerve stimulation can evoke emotional and energetic releases during the practice of Yoga.

This image illustrates the fascial planes and their movement in Urdhva Mukha Svanasana.

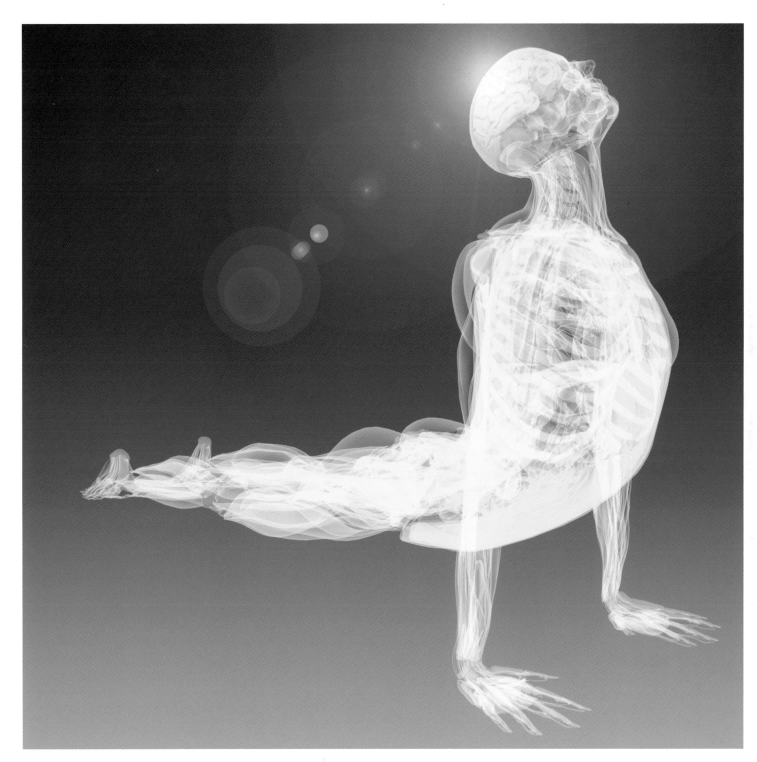

Chapter24
The Breath Connection

Regions of the brain, such as the brainstem, are highly evolved for survival; they control such complex functions as respiration with speed and precision that is far beyond comprehension by the conscious mind. Great instinctive power is stored in these regions of the brain. Hatha Yogic breathing techniques "yoke" or connect the conscious mind to the primal instinctive regions of the brainstem.

Athletes and martial arts practitioners access the breath's primal force by timing moments of exertion with forced exhalation. Yogis refine this by coordinating the rhythm of the breath with movements in the Asanas, generally coupling inhalation with expansion and exhalation with deepening. Pranayama perfects this process.

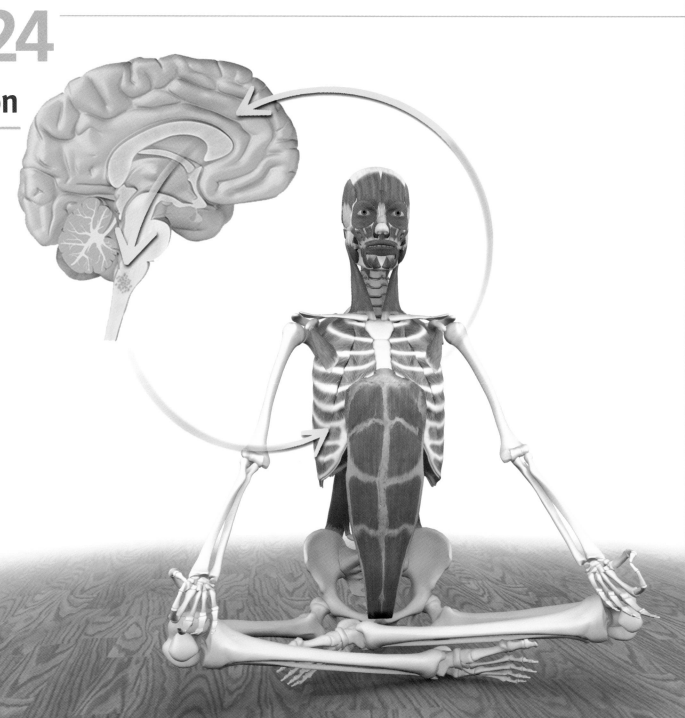

Inhalation and Exhalation

The diaphragm is the prime mover for inhalation and exhalation. It is a thin half-dome shaped muscle that separates the thoracic abdominal cavities. Contracting the diaphragm expands the chest, creating a negative inspiratory pressure in the thorax, and drawing air into the lungs through the trachea. Contracting the diaphragm also gently massages the abdominal organs.

Unlike most other skeletal muscles, the diaphragm rhythmically contracts and relaxes under the control of the autonomic nervous system, via the phrenic nerve. We are unaware of the diaphragm, unless we consciously think about its function.

Yogic breathing techniques such as Pranayama involve consciously contracting the diaphragm and controlling the breathing, thereby connecting the conscious and unconscious mind.

These images demonstrate the diaphragm contracting and relaxing. The lungs are elastic and expand when the diaphragm contracts during inhalation. Like a balloon, the lungs passively empty during exhalation as the diaphragm relaxes.

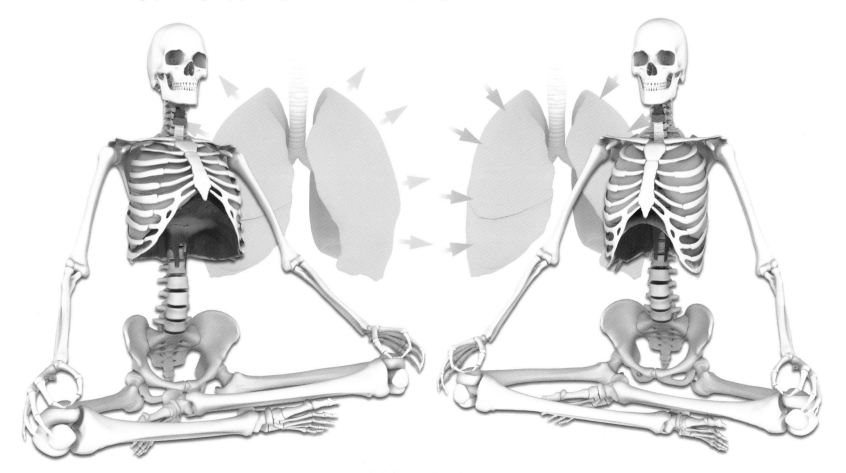

Ujayi Breath

When we breathe, the air passes through the nasal sinuses and pharynx into the trachea and into the lungs, oxygenating the blood and removing carbon dioxide. The pharynx and nasal passages are lined with blood-rich mucosa. The nasal sinuses create turbulence, increasing the amount of air contacting the mucosa. This process warms the air before it passes into the lower parts of the respiratory tract.

The glottis is a muscular aperture below the pharynx and nasal passages. Opening and closing the glottis regulates the flow of air into the lower respiratory tract. Normally we control the opening and closing of the glottis unconsciously.

Yogic breathing techniques involve consciously regulating airflow through the glottis. For example, we seal the glottis when performing Nauli so that the negative inspiratory pressure generated by contracting the diaphragm draws the abdominal contents upward instead of drawing breath into the trachea.

Consciously narrowing the opening of the glottis increases the turbulence of the air passing through the nasal and pharyngeal cavities. This action increases the transfer of heat to the air from the blood-rich mucosal lining, raising the temperature of the air above normal. Increasing air turbulence also creates an audible vibration similar to that of a flame leaping up from a fire. This process of increasing heat and creating vibration with the air is known as Ujayi breathing and is fundamental to the practice of Pranayama or "Breath of Fire."

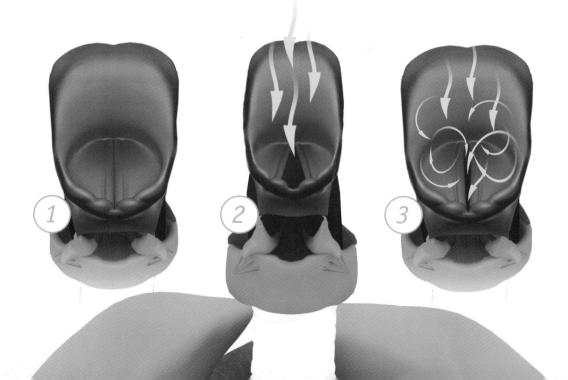

Accessory Muscles of Breath

Accessing the force of the accessory muscles of breath expands the lung volume and increases the turbulence of air in the respiratory passageways. As with postural muscles, we are generally not conscious of these accessory breath muscles until awakening them consciously. Focusing on contracting these muscles brings them under conscious control with profound effects. The following pages illustrate this process in Siddhasana, Virabhadrasana II, Tadasana and Uttanasana.

Thoracic Bellows

Begin awakening the accessory muscles of breath by drawing the scapulae toward the midline. Hold this position and then attempt to roll the shoulders forward by contracting the pectoralis minor. This closed-chain contraction lifts and opens the lower ribcage like a bellows and expands the lung volume.

Begin by practicing in Siddhasana, and then apply this technique to other postures, such as twists, that constrict the volume of the thoracic cavity.

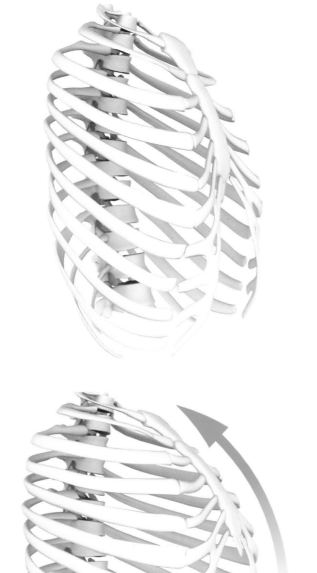

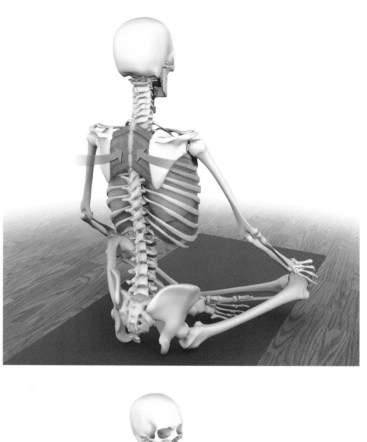

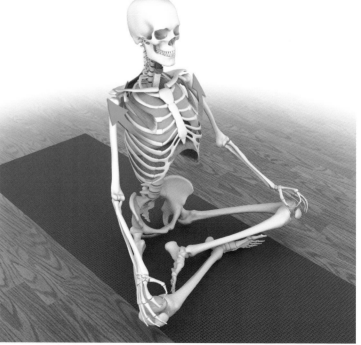

Accessory Muscles of Breath

1) Straighten the lower back by contracting the erector spinae and quadratus lumborum. This draws the lower posterior ribcage downward.

2) Balance this action by gently contracting the rectus abdominis. This draws the lower anterior ribcage downward and compresses the abdominal organs against the diaphragm, dynamizing its contraction and strengthening it.

3) Draw the shoulder blades together by contracting the rhomboids. This opens the front of the chest.

4) Maintain the contraction of the rhomboids and simultaneously contract the pectoralis minor and sternocleidomastoid. This lifts and opens the ribcage like a bellows.

Complete this process by pressing the hands down on the knees to fully open the chest (by contracting the latissimus dorsi).

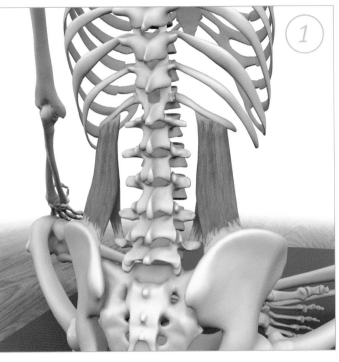
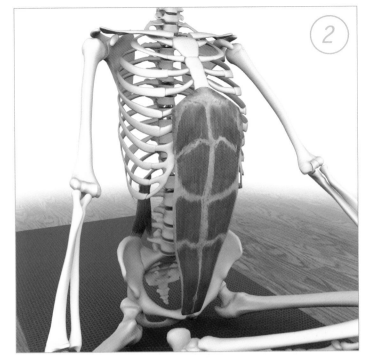
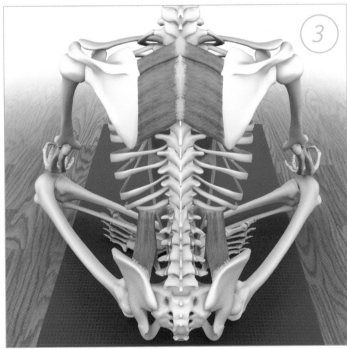
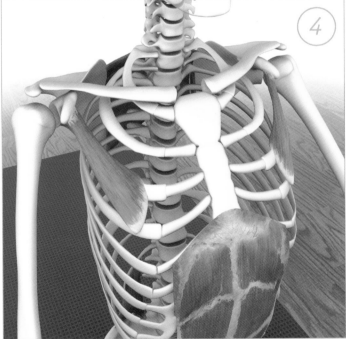

Exhalation

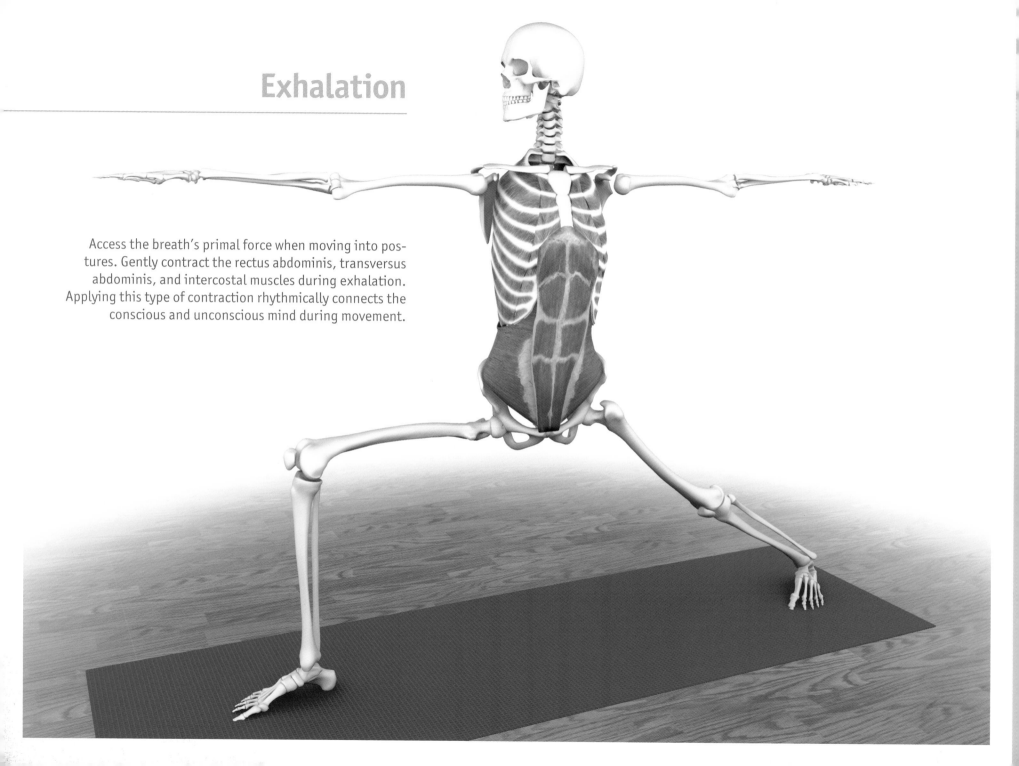

Access the breath's primal force when moving into postures. Gently contract the rectus abdominis, transversus abdominis, and intercostal muscles during exhalation. Applying this type of contraction rhythmically connects the conscious and unconscious mind during movement.

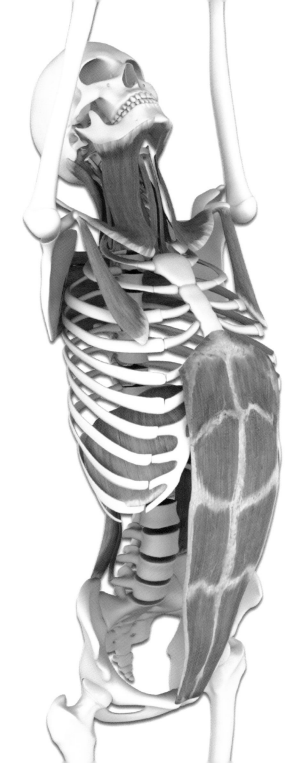

Synergy

Train the accessory breathing muscles so that they work synergistically to expand and contract the thorax during movement.

Increase the lung volume during inhalation by contracting the accessory breathing muscles in various combinations. For example, combine the rhomboids with the pectoralis minor, or the rectus abdominis with the quadratus lumborum (illustrated here in Tadasana).

Expel the residual air in the lungs during exhalation by contacting the rectus abdominis, transversus abdominis, and intercostal muscles.

Awakening the accessory breathing muscles is an extremely powerful technique. Begin with very gentle contraction and progress slowly and with great care. Never force any Yoga technique, especially breathing. Always proceed with caution under the guidance of an instructor.

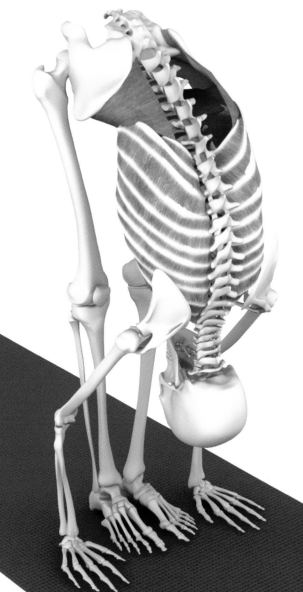

Chapter 25
Bandhas

Bandhas are "locks" occuring throughout the body. The combination of opposing muscles forms these "locks," stimulating nerve conduction and illuminating the Chakras.

Mula Bandha

Mula Bandha contracts the muscles of the pelvic floor, lifting and toning the organs of the pelvis, including the bladder and genitalia. The pelvic floor muscles are recruited and awakened by contracting associated muscles, such as the iliopsoas. This focuses the mind on the first Chakra.

Simultaneously contracting other muscle groups accentuates Mula Bandha. For example, gently squeezing the knees together (by contracting the adductors) increases contraction of the pelvic floor muscles. Pressing the hands together has the same effect. This phenomenon is known as "recruitment."

Udyana Bandha

Udyana Bandha contracts the upper abdominals located approximately two inches below the solar plexus and focuses the mind on the third Chakra.

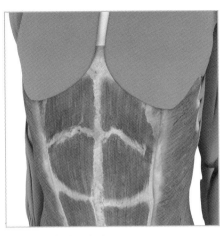

rectus abdominis

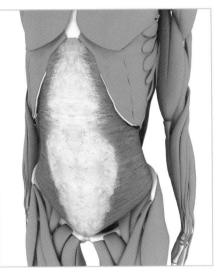

transversus abdominus

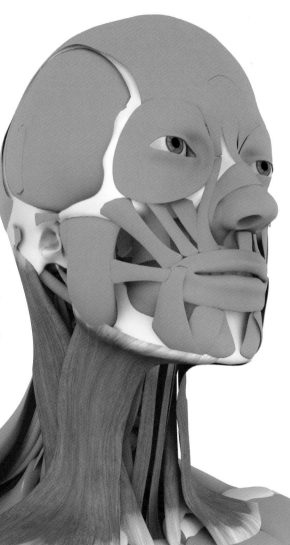

Jalandhara Bandha

Jalandhara Bandha contracts the anterior neck muscles, flexing the neck and drawing the chin to the sternum. This focuses the mind on the fifth Chakra.

Chapter26

Chakras

The Chakras are the subtle energy centers of the body. Like pinwheels, the Chakras spin at the speed of light, emanating the colors of the spectrum, each resonating with a particular frequency. These colors combine to form the auras that surround each of us, connecting us with each other and with the cosmos.

There are seven to eight major and numerous minor Chakras in the body. Their locations correspond to regions of the body where nerves collect and electrical activity is high, such as the brachial and sacral plexi (major Chakras) and the elbows and knees (minor Chakras).

The flow of energy in the Chakras can become blocked by life events through the activity of the autonomic nervous system. For example, when we habitually assume a defensive posture in response to negative stimuli, we block the flow of energy in the Chakras. Hatha Yoga counteracts this and re-illuminates the Chakras, stimulating them to spin freely.

Kundalini awakening refers to the "unblocking" of the flow of energy through and between the Chakras. This process can occur instantaneously from contact with a master (inner or outer) who awakens the student's awareness of his or her potential. Classically, this occurs through a touch but can occur with a glance or even through the mere presence of the master. This is known as Shak-tipata (the transmission of psycho-spiritual energy). As human consciousness transitions from the Piscean to the Aquarian Age, more and more people are spontaneously experiencing varying degrees of Kundalini awakening.

Kundalini awakening is akin to tapping into a high-voltage line and requires careful preparation. Hatha Yoga prepares the practitioner and awakens the Kundalini at the same time.

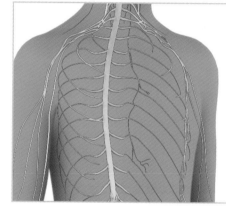

brachial plexus

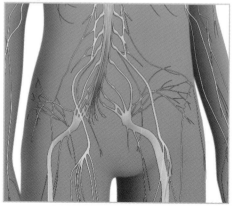

sacral plexus

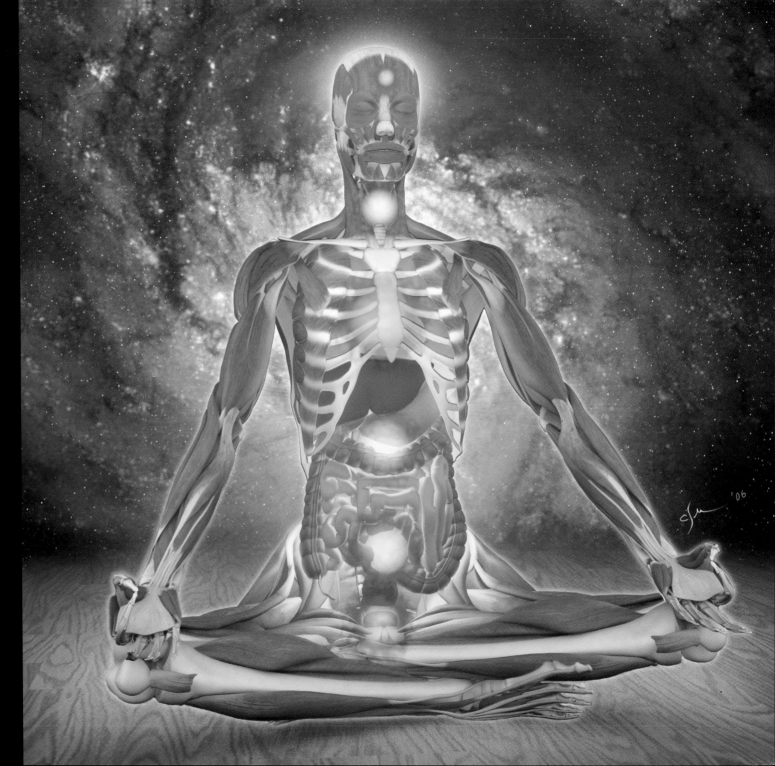

Asanas connect the body and mind. Breathing techniques connect the conscious and the unconscious. Chakra meditation connects the individual to the vibrational energy of the cosmos. Spend a few moments gazing at this image of the Chakras and then meditate as you visualize them. The Chakras will appear as a subtle but scintillating light within you.

Putting It All
Together

Balance all of the forces acting throughout the musculoskeletal system. Contract, relax, and stretch the appropriate muscles, and the bones will align themselves automatically. Synergistically combine the Asanas to complete the process (discussed in Scientific Keys, Volume II).

This sequence illustrates the process of combining muscles sequentially in lunge pose:

1. Position the body in lunge pose to begin stretching the iliopsoas.

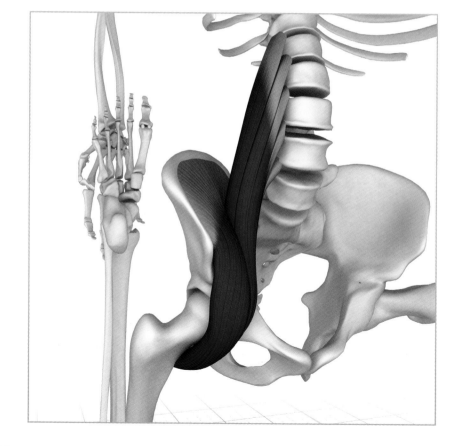

2. Contract the front leg hamstrings, drawing the body deeper into the lunge, accentuating the iliopsoas stretch.

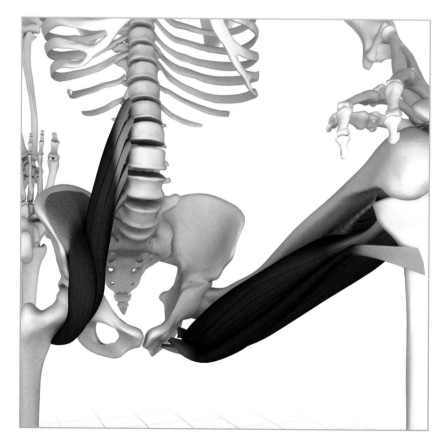

3. Contract the back arm biceps to flex the back knee, further accentuating the iliopsoas stretch (and stretching the quadriceps).

4. Contract the front arm triceps, straightening the arm and lifting the chest. This stretches the rectus abdominis, tilting the pelvis backward, and completing the iliopsoas stretch.

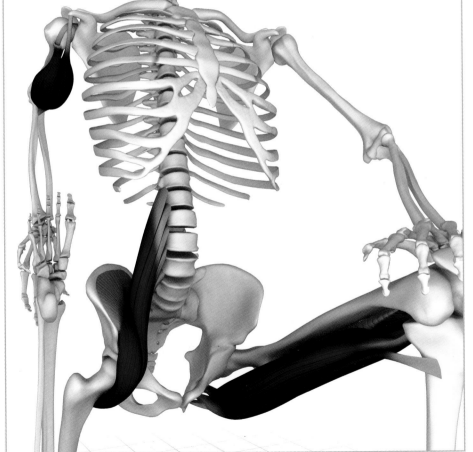

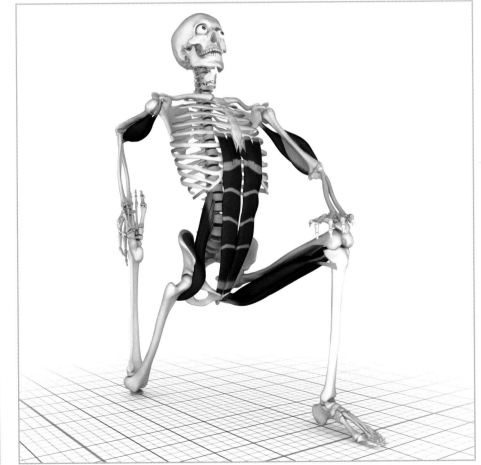

Easing into Downward Dog

1) This image illustrates Downward Facing Dog pose with tight hamstrings. Note how the pull of the hamstrings tilts the pelvis backwards (retroversion). This pulls the lumbosacral fascia and back muscles, so that the lower back loses some of its natural arch.

2) Bend the knees to release the hamstings and free the lower back. Contract the iliopsoas to tilt the pelvis forward (anteversion). This action brings back the natural arch of the lower back and draws the trunk toward the thighs.

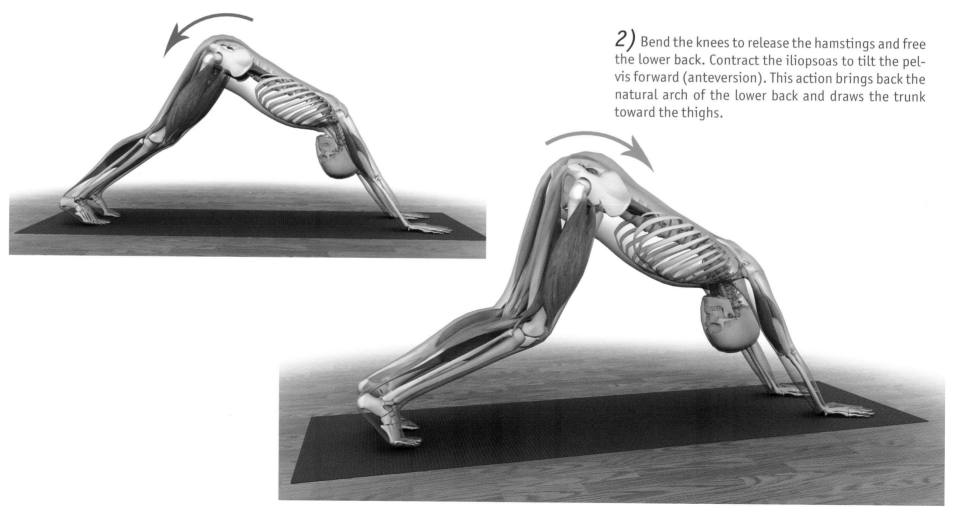

3) Contract the triceps to straighten the elbows.

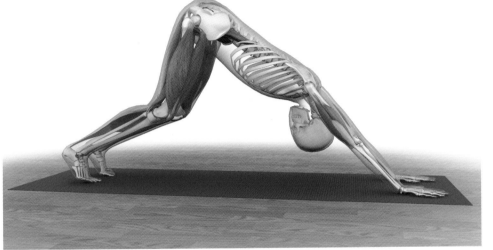

4) Maintain the contraction of the ilopsoas to fix the pelvis in anteversion. Then contract the quadriceps to straighten the knees and draw the hamstrings out to full stretch, completing the pose.

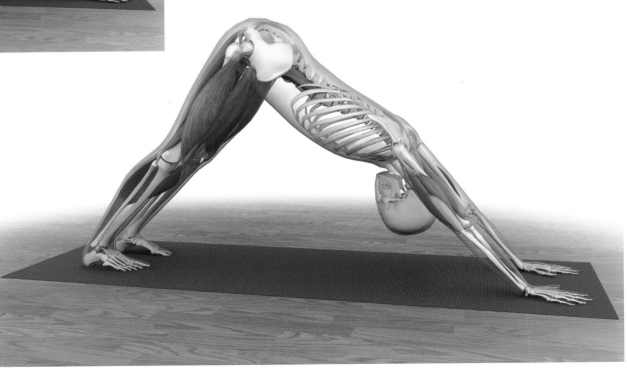

Optimizing Siddhasana

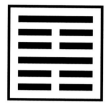

The ancient Chinese oracle, the I-Ching, contains fundamental instruction for the practice of Yoga in the hexagram "Keeping Still" (52 Kên). This hexagram resembles a vertebral unit of the spine. The text contains instruction for achieving stillness by stabilizing the spine from the sacrum to the skull.

This section shows how to optimize Siddhasana by sequentially activating various muscles, as follows:

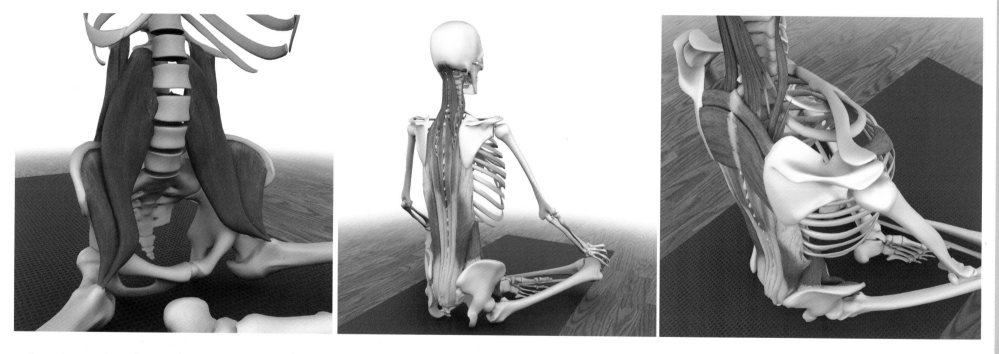

1) Contract the psoas and quadratus lumborum to stabilize the lumbosacral spine and ground the pelvis.

2) Contract the erector spinae to straighten the spine and move energy upward.

3) Draw the scapulae toward the midline by contracting the rhomboids. This action opens the chest. Balance this by closed-chain contraction of the pectoralis minor to lift the ribcage.

Optimizing Siddhasana

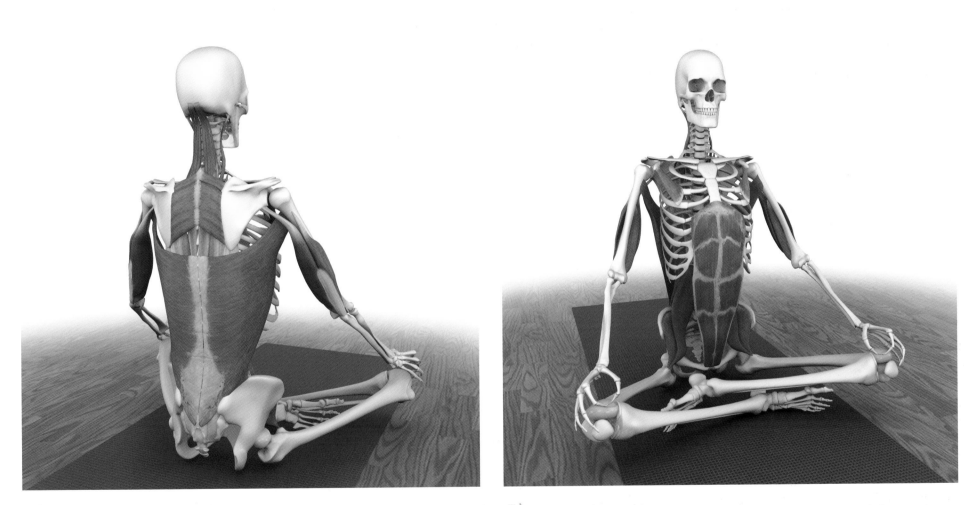

4) Contract the latissimus dorsi to further open the chest. Lift the spine by gently contracting the triceps, pressing the hands into the knees.

5) Complete and balance the pose by adding the rectus abdominis to activate Udyana Bandha.

Appendix of Asanas

Adho Mukha Svanasana
Downward Dog Pose

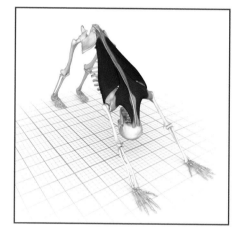

Adho Mukha Vrksasana
Full Arm Balance

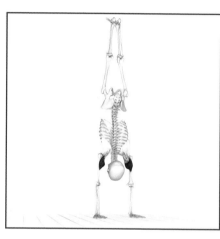

Ardha Chandrasana
Half Moon Pose

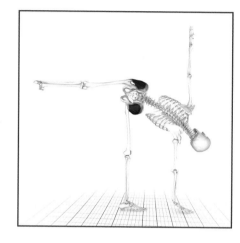

Baddha Konasana
Bound Angle Pose

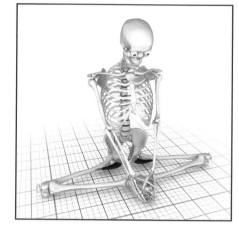

Bakasana
Crow Pose

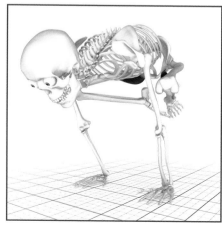

Chataranga Dandasana
Four Limb Staff Pose

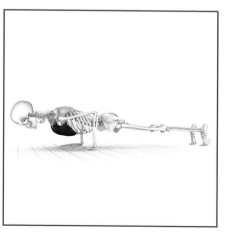

Danurasana
Bow Pose

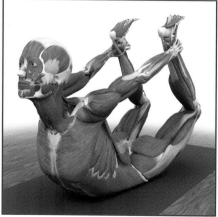

Eka Pada Viparita Dandasana
One Legged Inverted Staff Pose

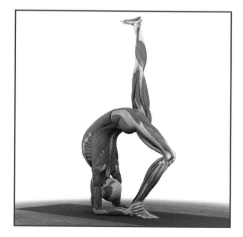

Garudasana
Eagle Pose

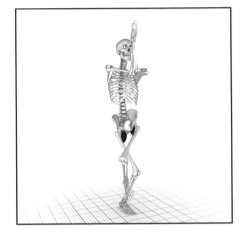

Gomukhasana B
Cow's Face Pose

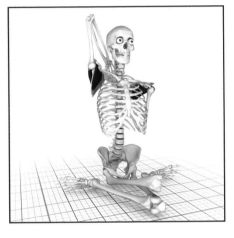

Janu Sirsasana
Head-to-Knee Pose

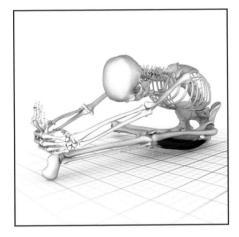

Kurmasana
Turtle Pose

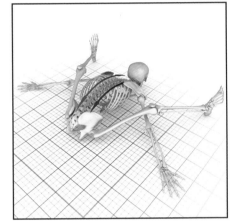

Marichyasana I
Sage Pose

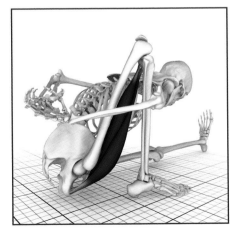

Marichyasana III
Sage Pose

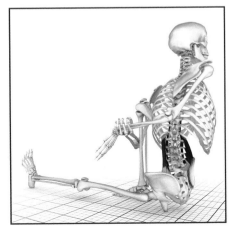

Navasana
Boat Pose

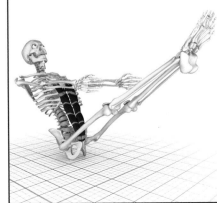

Padmasana
Lotus Pose

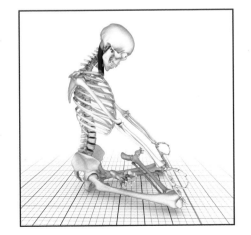

Appendix of Asanas

Supta Padangusthasana B
Sleeping Big Toe Pose

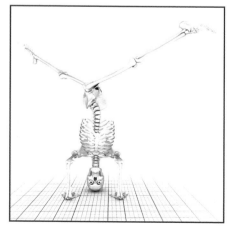

Utthita Hasta Padangusthasana
Great Toe Pose

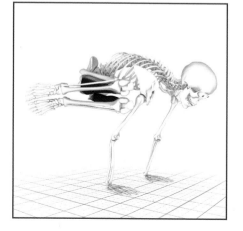

Parivrtta Trikonasana
Revolving Triangle Pose

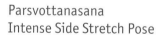
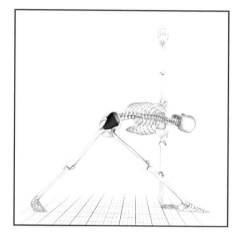

Parivrtta Parsvakonasana
Revolving Side Angled Pose

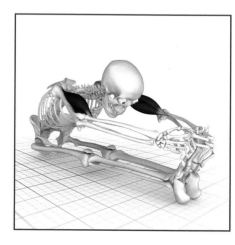

Parivrttaikapada Sirasana
Revolved Headstand Pose

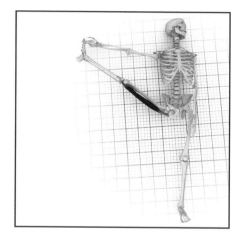

Parsva Bakasana
Revolved Crow Pose

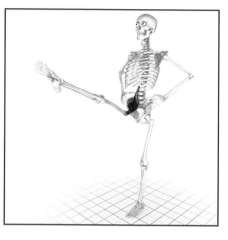

Parsvottanasana
Intense Side Stretch Pose

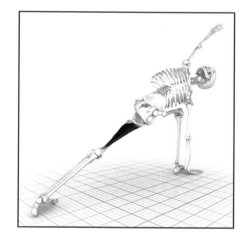

Paschimottanasana
Intense Stretch to the West Pose

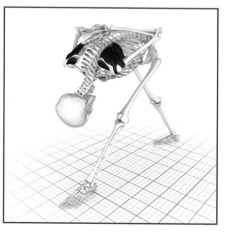

Prasarita Padottanasana
Wide Feet Intense Stretch Pose

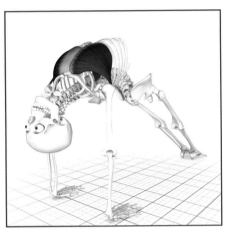

Purvottanasana
Intense Stretch to the East Pose

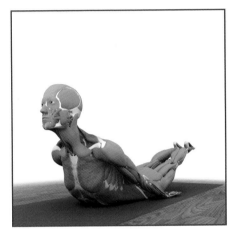

Salabhasana
Locust

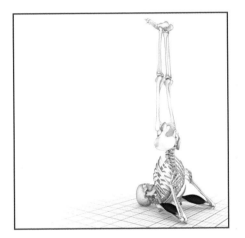

Sarvangasana
Shoulder Stand

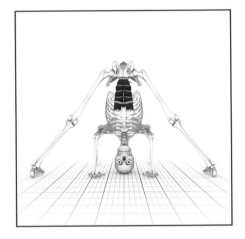

Setubandha Sarvangasana
Bridge Pose

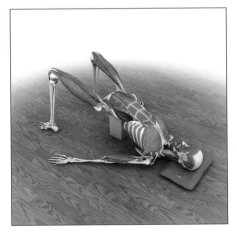

Siddhasana
The Seer Pose

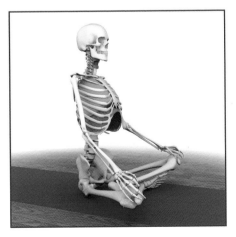

Supta Padangusthasana
(Bent Knee Version)

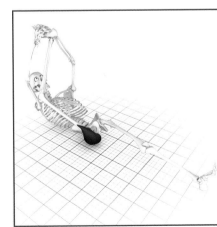

Urdhva Hastasana
Mountain Pose

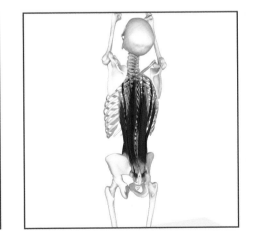

Appendix of Asanas

Tolasana
Scale Pose

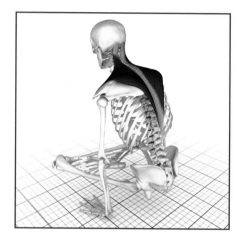

Upavistha Konasana
Seated Wide Angle

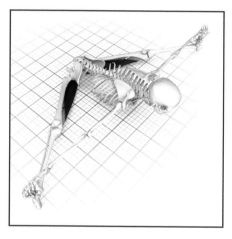

Urdhva Mukha Svanasana
Upward Facing Dog Pose

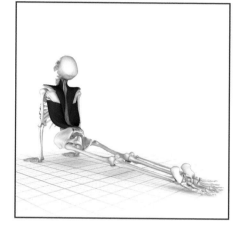

Urdhva Danurasana
Upward Bow

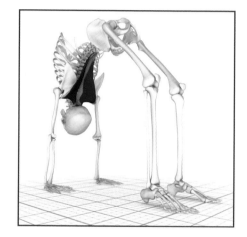

Ustrasana
Camel Pose

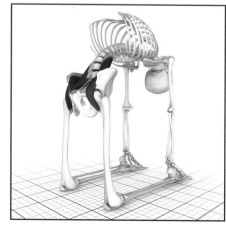

Utkatasana
Chair Pose

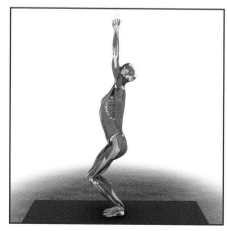

Uttanasana
Intense Forward Bending Pose

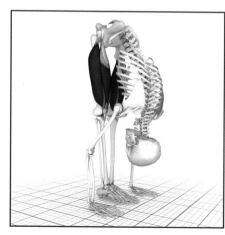

Utthita Trikonasana
Triangle Pose

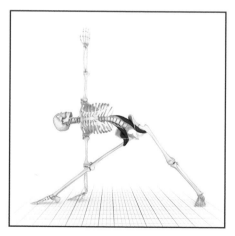

Vatayanasana
Horse Face Pose

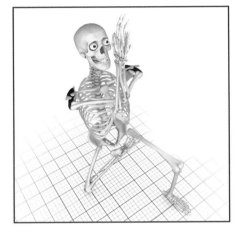

Virabhadrasana I
Warrior I

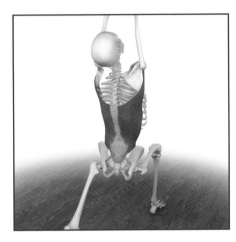

Virabhadrasana II
Warrior II

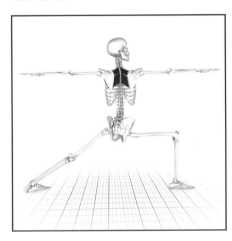

Virabhadrasana III
Warrior III

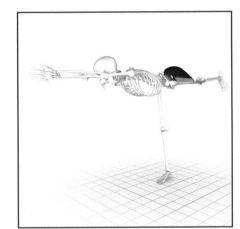

Vrishchikasana
Scorpion Pose

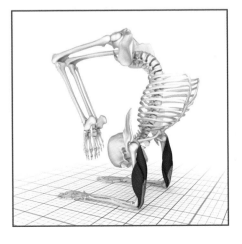

Vrksasana
Tree Pose

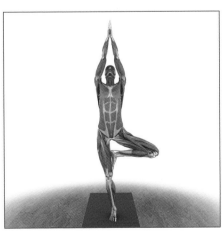

Index of Asanas

Index of Muscles

Also from Bandha Yoga

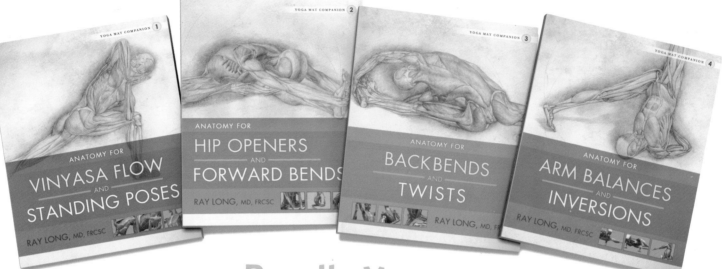

www.BandhaYoga.com

Your resource for anatomy and Yoga on the Web!

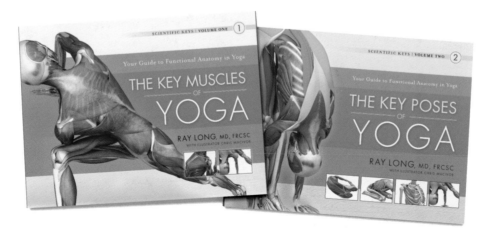